Disability and the University

Disability and the University

A Disabled Students' Manifesto, 2nd Edition

Christopher McMaster and Benjamin Whitburn, Editors

With a Foreword by Mike Oliver

Foreword to the Second Edition by Tanya Titchkosky & Rod Michalko

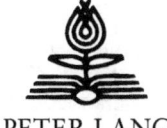

PETER LANG
New York · Berlin · Bruxelles · Chennai · Lausanne · Oxford

Library of Congress Cataloging-in-Publication Data

Names: McMaster, Christopher (Christopher Todd), editor. | Whitburn, Ben, editor.
Title: Disability and the university: a disable students' manifesto / Christopher McMaster, Benjamin Whitburn.
Description: Second edition. | New York: Peter Lang, 2025. | Includes bibliographical references.
Identifiers: LCCN 2024042297 (print) | LCCN 2024042298 (ebook) | ISBN 9783034357814 (paperback) | ISBN 9783034357838 (pdf) | ISBN 9783034357821 (epub)
Subjects: LCSH: College students with disabilities. | College students with Disabilities–Political activity. | Inclusive education.
Classification: LCC LC4818.38 .D56 2025 (print) | LCC LC4818.38 (ebook) | DDC 378.0087–dc23/ENG/20241028
LC record available at https://lccn.loc.gov/2024042297
LC ebook record available at https://lccn.loc.gov/2024042298
DOI 10.3726/b22820

Bibliographic information published by the Deutsche Nationalbibliothek.
The German National Library lists this publication in the German National Bibliography; detailed bibliographic data is available on the Internet at http://dnb.d-nb.de.

Cover design by Peter Lang Group AG

ISBN 9783034357814 (paperback)
ISBN 9783034357838 (ebook)
ISBN 9783034357821 (epub)
DOI 10.3726/b22820

© 2025 Peter Lang Group AG, Lausanne
Published by Peter Lang Publishing Inc., New York, USA
info@peterlang.com - www.peterlang.com

All rights reserved.
All parts of this publication are protected by copyright.
Any utilization outside the strict limits of the copyright law, without the permission of the publisher, is forbidden and liable to prosecution.
This applies in particular to reproductions, translations, microfilming, and storage and processing in electronic retrieval systems.

This publication has been peer reviewed.

In remembrance of Mike Oliver

Table of Contents

Foreword to the First Edition — xi
    Mike Oliver

Foreword to the Second Edition — xiii
    Tanya Titchkosky & Rod Michalko

Chapter 1 Post-Pandemic Opportunities for Inclusion in Higher Education — 1
    Ben Whitburn and Christopher McMaster

Part I Is Inclusion Really Part of the Culture of the Academy?

Chapter 2 Cripping Time: Temporalities in Academia — 11
    Jentel Van Havermaet

Chapter 3 Slowness, Disability, and Academic Productivity: The Need to Rethink Academic Culture — 19
    Travis Chi Wing Lau

Chapter 4 Disability Advocacy Within the Ableist Environment of Academia — 29
    Denise Beckwith

Chapter 5 The Violent Consequences of Disclosure … and How Disabled and Mad Students Are Pushing Back   39
Fady Shanouda

Chapter 6 Negotiating the Space of Academia as a Disabled Student   49
Leechin Heng

Chapter 7 Disability Studies in Higher Education: Developing Identity and Community   59
Megan Zahneis

Part II Adjustments for Learning and Contributing

Chapter 8 Beyond Compliance: Disabled Student Activism on Campus   69
Justin Freedman, Laura Jaffee, Katie Roquemore, Yosung Song and Hetsie Veitch

Chapter 9 Reasonable Adjustments   79
George Low

Chapter 10 But You Look Fine: Limitations of the Letter of Accommodation   87
Zoie Sheets

Chapter 11 The Need for Systemic Supports: Barriers Faced by Students with Disabilities in the Majority World   95
Mostafa Attia

Chapter 12 A Hierarchy of Impairments: The Absence of Body Size in Disability Accommodations Within Universities   103
Erin Pritchard

Chapter 13 *"I Can't Even Reach the Waffle-Maker!"*: Increasing Access for Students with Physical Disabilities on University Campuses   111
April B. Coughlin

Chapter 14 Assistance Dogs and Academia: Supporting the Dynamic Duo in the post-COVID "New World"   121
Dr. G. Geller and Dr. A. Müller

Chapter 15 Universalizing International Exchange for Students with Disabilities   133
Justin Harford

Chapter 16 Creating an Accessible and Resilient Environment inside the Indian University   143
P. Boopathi and K. Muruganandan

Part III Getting Access, Asserting Rights

Chapter 17 If Not Now, When? Catalyzing Solidarity for Enduring Belonging in Higher Education   155
  Laura Yvonne Bulk and Neera R. Jain

Chapter 18 Disabled by Society: Knowing and Invoking Your Rights   167
  Katelin Anderson and Beth Rogers

Chapter 19 Identifying and Eliminating Digital Barriers after COVID   177
  Karen McCall

Chapter 20 Navigating the Mud of Tertiary Education: The Experience of Disabled Students at Universities in the Global South   189
  Tafadzwa Rugoho

Chapter 21 Even the Delusional Can Learn: The Recognition of Diverse States of Mind, Knowing and Being   197
  Maree Roche

Chapter 22 From Classification to Culture: Learning Disabilities in Higher Education   205
  Matthew Bereza

Chapter 23 Final Thoughts: Political Struggle in Higher Education   213
  Ben Whitburn and Christopher McMaster

Contributors   219

Foreword to the First Edition

MIKE OLIVER

In 2017 I returned to my old university to deliver an open lecture. I had spent many happy years there as an undergraduate, postgraduate and then lecturer in the 1970s and early 1980s. The changes I saw that day were surprising to say the least. There were new buildings and people everywhere and the campus seemed much larger and much busier than I had remembered it.

University life was much more relaxed when I turned up as an undergraduate in 1972. There were just over 5000 students on campus and throughout the 10 years I spent studying and working there I only met 4 other disabled students and one lecturer who used a wheelchair.

As a disabled wheelchair user back in 1972 I quickly found that the built environment of the campus made no concessions to my mobility needs; only one of the 4 colleges had a lift and there were no ramps, dropped kerbs or reserved parking spaces. Nor did I expect any at that time and I spent years being lifted to wherever I needed to go by fellow students. My life was made easier too by helpful porters, cleaners and catering staff willing to go the extra mile with help and support.

Additionally, no concessions were made to accessing the curriculum; there was no extra time in exams, no support staff working with disabled students and no information in other mediums. Such things simply did not exist at that time and there were no expectations that there should be from the authorities or students themselves.

During my recent visit there were more than 20,000 students on campus of whom more than 2,500 were disabled. There were many more buildings, built or being built often where green spaces used to be, and the campus was much more crowded with people rushing everywhere.

The growth I encountered on my return was very impressive and not just in size and numbers. The information and support currently available to disabled people wanting to study and work at the university was also remarkable. There was a Student Support & Wellbeing Team employing over 120 staff full and part-time, and they provided a whole range of services including educational support, mentoring, study skills tuition and support groups to students.

So where did this all come from? In my view there have been 2 main drivers. The first of these has been the sheer determination of increasing numbers of disabled people to access all of the things that non-disabled people for granted. All over the world disabled people have been coming together collectively and demanding that they be able to take their rightful place in the societies in which they live.

The second driver has been to place the experiences of disabled people centre stage both in developing economic and social policies generally and specifically opening up access to universities to all disabled people who wanted to study and work there. Facilitating this has been the development of disability studies as an academic discipline in its own right countering the individualistic and over-medicalised approaches which existed before.

But, of course, the changes noted above over the last 50 years couldn't have happened without the willingness of university authorities to accommodate all this. It would be wrong however to assume that nothing further needs to done and that all universities have become barrier free environments in the broadest sense of the term to all disabled people across the world. We should also note that global austerity policies have reversed some of the positive changes we have seen over the past fifty years.

This book makes a positive contribution to taking these changes into the future and hopefully reversing some of cuts already made or planned. It is based on the real-life experiences of those who have been there and done it. It also confronts outdated notions about what disabled people need and how best to prove it. Finally, it serves a guide to what needs to be done in the future so that, those looking back in 50 years time, will be as pleasantly surprised then as I am now about the changes that have taken place.

Mike Oliver
16/10/2018

Foreword to the Second Edition

TANYA TITCHKOSKY & ROD MICHALKO

We are sure of one thing: while the meaning of disability is structured in limited and limiting ways by the academy, disabled students are always more and other than these meanings and structures make them to be. Living precariously on this more than/less than precipice of academic life, disabled students represent the occasion and possibility for critical engagement with all forms of institutional life in contemporary culture. Disabled students do, after all, embody the cultural contradictions that flow from the more than/less than life of disability, contradictions that disabled students paradoxically also challenge.

We too have lived in precarity on this precipice and in the midst of these cultural contradictions. Both of us are disabled (Tanya is dyslexic and Rod is blind) and both of us live our disabilities in the academy; first, as students and then as faculty. Interestingly enough, our experiences as disabled students were eerily close to that of students today, that is, the academy did not expect us to show up.

But, there we were, representing the coming together of disability and the academy. This meant that sometimes faculty and administrators, other students, and even ourselves, came to know that life with disability in the academy was both more and less than we all first thought. What is intriguing for us, is that we did not expect that our particular interwoven experiences of blindness and dyslexia, and the general ways disability was made meaningful, would or could play such a predominant role in our scholarly research and teaching. Nor did we expect that this role would remain a definitive feature of life with disability in the academy and one which we, alongside disabled students, continue to respond to in myriad ways.

This *Disabled Students' Manifesto* is a lively testimony to these many responses. And yet, the university continues to excel in generating limited and limiting conceptions of disability as a problem to be solved, as an unwanted condition to be detected, managed, and even eradicated. Curiously, this continues in the academy in the midst of the sentiment expressed in the oft used phrase, "we've come a long way, but there is a long way to go." Nonetheless, disabled students tenaciously remain, in Paul Hunt's (1998 [1966], p. 18) terms, an "uncomfortable, subversive ... living reproach to any scale of values" that conceives disability as only a problem to be solved, as merely objects of research. As a disruption to the dominant social imaginary of the normative order, disabled students continue to show how the academy needs to struggle to realize that disability offers a form of perception. Disabled students show, too, that disability can potentially offer a generative and even new understanding of the normative order and show how disability is needed in that order, including that of the academy.

Despite the increase in the number of disabled students, faculty and staff on university campuses, as Mike Oliver highlighted in his Foreword to the first edition of this volume, the academy stubbornly clings to its exclusive orientation toward disability. Our discipline of sociology, for example, participates greedily in this dominant social imaginary that significantly restricts the meaning of disability. Sociology typically frames disability as either a form of deviance (usually involuntary) or as the added-on lesser variable within the gender, class, race tri-factor. Framed this way, knowledge of adaptation, passing, or social control of disabled people is generated but knowledge of disability as a life-worth-living, as a way of perceiving, knowing and being, remains beyond the scope of the sociological "eye."

Since the 1981 International Year of Disabled Persons, it has become more and more common for disabled people to be included as *anticipated participants* in society, including in the academy. The proliferation of university policies and procedures in relation to the accommodation of disability attests to this anticipated participation. These policies and procedures, which are now global, typically emphasize the student as responsible for any accommodation they might require. It is the student who is tasked with seeking out the office charged with accommodation. It is the student who is tasked with proving that they are legitimately disabled thus deserving of services. Anticipated is one thing, expected is another matter altogether.

Anticipated but not expected: this is the current predicament for disabled people on our campuses. While surrounded by anticipatory structures of individualized accommodation, disabled students are met with educational practices, platforms, protocols and policies that still do not expect them to show up. The academy limits its conception and subsequent engagement with disability to a matter of "fit." Disabled students who do not easily fit are, therefore, not easily accommodated whereas those students conceived of by the academy as "easy-fits" are easily accommodated. This demonstrates why university admission platforms and student recruitment strategies are rarely touched by disability-friendly practices.

The second edition of *A Disabled Students' Manifesto* raises many important questions in the midst of the COVID-19 pandemic, a phenomenon that re-ordered university life. Did structural responses to pandemic protocols change not only forms of access and accommodation but also forms of meaning for disabled students? Have disabled students been recognized as more and other than an unexpected but bureaucratically anticipated problem population? Has the University awakened to its need for disabled students and disability studies for its own well-being? *A Disabled Students' Manifesto* helps us to engage these questions and raises many more. It encourages us to think about the scales of value and the forms of knowledge that are organizing our lives together in all our academic relations, through COVID-19 pandemic measures and well beyond.

Questions of accessibility and accommodation might be understood as the beginning point for re-engaging the limited and limiting ways the university engages disabled students. What is required is for all of us to consider, now that we might find our way into the academy, what remains for us as disabled people beyond anticipated access procedures. What difference can and should disability now make?

REFERENCE

Hunt, P. (1998 [1966]). A critical condition. In T. Shakespeare (Ed.), *The disability reader: Social science perspectives* (pp. 1–19). London: Cassell.

CHAPTER 1

Post-Pandemic Opportunities for Inclusion in Higher Education

BEN WHITBURN AND CHRISTOPHER McMASTER

INTRODUCTION

Political struggle is what has led to people with disabilities gaining access to higher education institutions worldwide. We hold fast to this institutional memory—and this is indeed how we started the previous edition of this edited volume (McMaster & Whitburn, 2019), which we dedicated to the late Mike Oliver, who contributed, as far as we know, his final piece of writing. As Oliver himself acknowledged, the effect of this political struggle is evident through the increased enrolments universities around the world have received involving students disclosing disabilities (read also Hubble & Bolton, 2021; Pittman & Brett, 2022). Yet, we must also acknowledge that today, inclusion in higher education for students with disabilities has been sorely tested at the height of the global COVID-19 pandemic, revealing cracks in the established infrastructure (if such a polity existed at all) in support of such participation. With mandated lockdowns gripping the world to encourage (and in some instances to mandate) social isolation, institutions of higher education quickly ramped up their reliance on technology for teaching and learning activities. For some universities, this presented a troubling adaptation from traditional face-to-face teaching; while others, particularly in wealthy global north contexts, pivoted easily to technology-mediated methods.

Students with disabilities may have been included in the hurried digitisation of learning when the COVID-19 pandemic hit—there was little choice. Yet, equity within the sector may have lasting negative effects (NEON, 2021); but we might also hope for more affirming ones. It was precisely this issue that triggered the formation of this second edition of the manifesto, in which we maintain and reinforce the significance of an approach to disability studies that emphasises the experiences of students with disabilities, while at the same time thinking about the new post-pandemic opportunities for inclusion in higher education that will undoubtedly emerge. Here we will touch on three relevant points to this end: institutional efforts to support disabled students during COVID 19; the experiences of students in relation to such support; and the necessary advancement of inclusion in the sector beyond participation in a post-pandemic world.

INSTITUTIONAL EFFORTS TO SUPPORT STUDENTS WITH DISABILITIES DURING THE HEIGHT OF COVID-19

Universities in some countries claimed to have undertaken specific efforts to support students with disabilities to adapt to online learning at the height of the global COVID-19 pandemic. Take the UK as a case in point. Disability service managers were reportedly included in university-wide emergency response teams for most institutions in Britain from the commencement of lockdown measures, ensuring matters of access and support affecting students with disabilities were addressed systemically (National Association of Disability Practitioners [NAPD], 2021). As the NAPD report makes clear, as disability is not a homogenous category, students with different impairments were accordingly not all impacted in the same way. Nevertheless, consistently at stake was the capacity for education providers to continue to make reasonable adjustments for students with disabilities under the relevant legislation, while ensuring accessibility to key learning materials, including appropriate resourcing to ensure students could study from their homes.

Of course, assuring the upkeep of inclusive learning for disabled students as physical university campuses closed down was not an easy proposition: the shift to digitally-mediated learning was hurriedly implemented, leaving many disabled students in its wake, and further entrenching the individualised manner by which their inclusion in higher education is generally framed (Titchkosky, 2022; Thomas & Whitburn, in print). In South Africa, similar shortfalls have been reported in comparison to the UK experience (Ntombela, 2022; Dube & Baleni, 2022), correlated principally with the ways universities compartmentalise support for students with disabilities as an add on to be provided by a particular office and specialist staff, rather than as a responsibility shared across institutional members. By these accounts, it seems likely that any systemic intent to maintain support for students with disabilities to ensure their ongoing success in higher education was lacking at the peak of the lockdown measures.

THE EXPERIENCES OF STUDENTS IN RELATION TO SUPPORT PROVISION

We make the last point hastily of course—in keeping with the conceptual orientations of this book, it would of course be wise to explore how students with disabilities themselves encountered the conditions of support that maintained their connection to higher education through the hurried transition to online-only learning. Once again in the UK—though we recognise it is a big world—the newly formed Disabled Students' Commission surveyed students across the Kingdom to learn of their experiences (Advanced HE, 2021). Of 473 respondents, the survey revealed that nearly 75% of commencing students felt their transition to higher education was adversely impacted by online learning measures, and just over 36% struggled to adapt to online learning. More than half expressed concerns about gaining employment after graduation, and over 80% indicated heightened mental health concerns due to these measures.

While it might be simple to discount Advance HE's (2021) survey results on sheer numbers alone—the survey scarcely reached a minor percentage of identified students with disability attending UK institutions of higher education, and Britain certainly does not represent a universal global view. These conclusions suggest that not all students with disabilities were adversely impacted by institutional responses to COVID-19. This resonates with other studies in different country contexts (Dube & Baleni, 2022; Wilson, L. et al, 2021; Wertans & Burch, 2022) that importantly explore the experiences of students with disabilities, and highlight the valuable contribution that flexibility to teaching, assessment, and the sensitivity of teaching and administration staff to their requirements, made to their sense of inclusive participation. All these studies share a particularity in common: they recommend higher education uphold a flexible approach to blended learning opportunities in the aftermath of COVID-19. Rather than simply adding to this chorus and hoping the sector takes note, we lay out a few suggestions to this end in the next section, to which new chapters in this second edition of the book reinforce.

STRUCTURE OF THE BOOK

Disability and the University: A Students' Manifesto is divided into three parts, each examining crucial aspects of further education, including the culture of the academy, moving beyond the limits of compliance, access to and in the institution, and disability rights.

The remainder of Part I examines the culture of the academy—a culture that can exclude many by its very design. Privilege is a term explored widely in social research (Apple et al., 2010)—privilege in a culture that can exclude by overt and implicit design. The chapters in this section consider what it means to navigate this culture, and in so doing considers how it can be changed.

In Chapter 2, Jentel Van Havermaet takes up one of the underlying (though not frequently scrutinised) issues implicated in the education of people of all ages who live with disabilities: that of time, or crip time. In advancing the argument that students of higher education with disabilities ought not be expected to conform with stringent temporal frameworks as set by universities, Van Havermaet draws on personal experiences across a variety of different study-related tasks to demonstrate how time is contingently lived through disability. The take home message here is that time can also be understood and relational, and suggestions are given as to how that may be embedded in practice.

In Chapter 3, and also focused on time, Travis Chi Wing Lau presents a discussion of how both students and scholars with disabilities are excluded by the dominant temporal regimes of American neoliberal universities. Weaving theoretical understandings of the temporal and disability with an account of the frenetic pace of course requirements and assessment regimes, Lau takes solace from the slow academic movement to advocate for cultural change in universities. Lau's take-home message is that inclusion is affected by much more than mere admission to higher education programs.

In Chapter 4, Denise Beckwith addresses the ableism intrinsic to university processes, which require that ongoing, medically-based explanations are provided in order to attain reasonable adjustments to study. Beckwith demonstrates that in spite of a university's best intentions, lack of training can lead staff to neglect their responsibilities to provide safety and protection to all students. Beckwith portends the value of individual and collective advocacy for redressing entrenched notions of integration over inclusion.

In a similar vein, Chapter 5 is presented by Fady Shanouda on the complex terrain of disclosure in higher education. Shanouda describes processes of both formal and informal disclosure of one's condition as institutional violence that leads to visceral consequences. Shanouda advocates for the formation of alliances with critically-oriented university staff as a way of finding comfort through a person's studies.

Leechin Heng's contribution occupies Chapter 6, in which she considers how knowledge about disability is taken for granted in higher education providers, and as well in their course programs. Implicit rules position students with disabilities in particular ways, which can and do go by unchallenged. Heng suggests ways that higher education providers can break this mould by actively working with diverse worldviews, in particular of those with disabilities.

Chapter 7 concludes the first section of the book in which Megan Zahneis turns her attention to the role of higher education study in the formation of students' identities. To this end, higher education institutions have a significant role in supporting people with disabilities in affirming their identities—a portentous message given the discussions presented in the preceding chapters of the book. Zahneis calls for the intentional inclusion of disability studies scholarship in course curricula, for the value it can provide to subjective wellbeing and self-understanding. She demonstrates the impact of disability studies curricula beyond the confines of the classroom, to processes core to an institution's culture.

Part II demands careful consideration beyond what is offered, beyond the limits of compliance, beyond letters of accommodation, and beyond what is considered, at this moment in time, as "reasonable accommodations." It asks the reader to consider their own power—achieving more rights through organization and activism, as a previous generation has done.

In Chapter 8, Justin Freedman, Laura Jaffee, Katie Roquemore, Yosung Song and Hetsie Veitch introduce readers to a committee deliberately set up at a university whose objective is to support the institution to go beyond mere compliance in its efforts to respond to demands for inclusivity. Disability studies inform committee activities, including mandatory training at the university and activist events. The authors demonstrate the significance of addressing inequalities for students with disability as a priority for developing inclusive environments.

George Low explores the necessity as well as the limitations of reasonable adjustments in Chapter 9. The reductive tendency of universities to categorise impairments with adjustment type, and as well poor communication between staff, can significantly impact the efficacy of modifications available to students with disabilities. Low advocates intentional collaboration to ensure that adjustments are tailored to student need, as a priority for building inclusion into institutional practices.

In Chapter 10, Zoie Sheets explores letters of accommodation as a mechanism for supporting a disabled student's access to learning. Letters of accommodation, Sheets explains, can be taken up in very different ways by different university staff, in effect providing further barriers to learning. Sheets advises ways for students to ensure accommodation requirements are understood by teaching staff, while clarifying that documented adjustment necessities alone cannot sufficiently develop inclusive opportunities in higher education.

In Chapter 11 Erin Pritchard examines physical barriers on university campuses. Normative standards, even those designed to provide universal access to all, can persist, and Prichard's discussion unpacks these concerns by way of apparent hierarchies of impairment. Examining the exclusionary nature of these norms, Prichard highlights the significance of access to aspects of the built environment as mundane as doorways, chairs and tables and their impact on genuine inclusiveness.

In Chapter 12, Mostafa Attia addresses higher education participation for students with disabilities in majority world contexts. Barriers persist in admissions processes, inconsistent support services, inaccessible resource provision, and rigid assessment procedures. Attia describes the importance of collective action to effect change, as a priority for developing inclusive higher education systems in majority world countries.

In Chapter 13, April B. Coughlin explores the necessity to advocate strongly for universities to provide basic physical access to their facilities. Just as important to accessible campus facilities is the provision of inclusive and accessible accommodation. Coughlin contends that though higher education providers tout their commitment to diversity and inclusion, separated and specialist provisions tend to shadow these ideals. Coughlin advises students with disabilities to take up creative ways of advocating for change, including the development of videos that demonstrate the personal cost of inaccessible facilities.

Based in Australia, Georgia Geller is joined by Amanda Müller in an updated Chapter 14 to provide a post-COVID 19 account of how universities are legally-bound to accept assistance dogs onto campuses (as they were beforehand), and importantly, how such supports were central to their experiences during the height of lockdowns. Here they lay out a number of key updates higher education institutions should make to ensure they are more inclusive of students who depend on assistance animals as significant aspects of their day-to-day experiences.

Justin Harford explores the world in Chapter 15 by way of the necessity to ensure that international study exchange programs are inclusive of students with disabilities. Recognising that barriers prevent the participation of underrepresented students in international exchange, Harford recommends designing disability access requirements into exchange programs from the beginning. In so doing, Harford points to an aspect of higher education study that may otherwise seem impossible to also be inclusive of students with disabilities.

Boopathi P. and Muruganandan K. conclude Part III in Chapter 16 by returning to the majority world context, and a description of the struggles to achieve inclusion of students with disabilities into higher education. The authors describe a policy initiative that although effective in increasing participation of disabled students in higher education, requires deliberate attention to be implemented in full. The authors make suggestions for strengthening this important resource, from admission through the design of teaching and learning activities, curriculum and assessment practices.

Parts Three considers the topic of access, going beyond the concept as explored in the previous sections. Part III has a particular focus on the physical environment from multiple perspectives.

In a new Chapter 17, Laura Bulk and Neera Jain look to a socially just future in higher education, taking stock along the way of the values that different ways of being and knowing have influenced the sector. While this certainly starts with embracing the contribution of disability epistemologies, it reaches also towards Indigenous knowledges and other marginalised wisdoms that emphasise interdependence, flexibility, and the fundamental goals of education. These authors set out a useful set of core questions that higher education practitioners at all levels ought ask themselves to critically reflect on their own contribution to the project of inclusive co-existence.

In Chapter 18, Katelin Anderson and Beth Rogers explore some of the challenges associated with reasonable adjustments to learning programs in higher education, citing conflicts in practices that can be exclusive for students with disabilities. In many cases disability rights legislation is in place to counter any such conflicts, and the authors recommend students with disabilities to familiarise themselves with these in order to be able to assert their position. The authors offer practical strategies for both students and institutions to exercise legislated inclusive practices.

Chapter 19 comprises an updated discussion, by Karen McCall, about the significance of digital inclusion that was unquestionably given emphasis during the height of the COVID-19 pandemic; some good, some bad, and some that will hopefully remain. McCall updates her already useful set of strategies to inform the development of inclusive policies and practices related to digital environments, to maximise accessibility for students with disabilities.

Tafadzwa Rugoho returns our attention to the majority world context in Chapter 20, describing the increase of higher education providers and barriers to participation for students with disabilities that include negative attitudes, limited course offerings, and physical and technological accessibility. Wholesale changes to university infrastructure is required to broaden the participation of disabled students. To this end, Rugoho makes practical suggestions for change to both students and institutions.

In Chapter 21 Maree Roche attends to higher education participation for students with psychosocial disabilities. With a high prevalence of students with anxiety and related mental health concerns entering higher education, Roche's well-timed exploration of institutional practices to support student learning explores the sporadic nature of these conditions on learning. Roche's analysis comprises strategic recommendations to support learning, including how to engage with supervisors, how to plan and write up work, and what to expect from institutions.

Matthew Bereza concludes the book in Chapter 22 with a contribution about participation in higher education for students with learning difficulties. Access to learning can be easily compromised when higher education providers neglect to support students with intellectual impairments, to which Bereza responds by calling for radical inclusion—a deeply political program of inclusive development.

Bereza's clarion call to higher education institutions is to develop dedicated resources to this endeavour.

REFERENCES

Apple, M. W., Ball, S. J., & Gandin, L. A. (Eds.). (2010). *The Routledge international handbook of the sociology of education*. New York, NY: Routledge.

Dube, N., & Baleni, L. (2022). The Experiences of Higher Education Students with Disabilities in Online Learning during the COVID-19 Pandemic. *Journal of Culture and Values in Education*, 5(1), 59–77.

Hubble, S., & Bolton, P. (2021). *Support for disabled students in higher education in England*. London, UK: House of Commons Library.

McMaster, C., & Whitburn, B. (2019). *Disability and the university: A disabled students' manifesto*. New York, NY: Peter Lang Publishing Group.

NEON, N. E. O. N. (2021). *Perspectives on the challenges to access and equity in higher Education across the world in the context of COVID* [Report]. W. A. t. H. E. D. (WAHED). https://worldaccesshe.com/wp-content/uploads/2021/09/SBT2369-National-Education-Opportunities-Network-NEON-Report-Design-v3-Single-Page.pdf

Ntombela, S. (2022). Reimagining South African higher education in response to Covid-19 and ongoing exclusion of students with disabilities. *Disability & Society*, 37(3), 534–539.

Pitman, T., & Brett, M. (2022). Disability and Australian higher education: The case for an Accessible model of disability support. *Australian Journal of Education*, 66(3), 314–325.

Thomas, M. K. E., & Whitburn, B. In *Review. 8 The Plague years in Higher Education* (M. Murphy, H. Moscovitz, M. Martini, & S. Robertson, Eds.). (2023). Building the Post-Pandemic University. London, UK: Edward Elgar Publishing.

Titchkosky, T. (2022). University Inclusion Practices–Re-Encountering the Status Quo: An Interpretive Approach. *Journal of Disability Studies in Education*, 3(1), 102–124.

Wertans, E., & Burch, L. (2022). 'It's Backdoor Accessibility': Disabled Students' Navigation of University Campus. *Journal of Disability Studies in Education*, 3(1), 57–78.

Wilson, L., Conway, N., Martin, N. and Turner, P. (2021). Covid-19: Disabled Students in Higher Education: Student Concerns and Institutional Challenges: Report by the National Association of Disability Practitioners. London, UK: National Association of Disability Practitioners (NAPD).

PART I

IS INCLUSION REALLY PART OF THE CULTURE OF THE ACADEMY?

CHAPTER 2

Cripping Time: Temporalities in Academia

JENTEL VAN HAVERMAET

INTRODUCTION: TEMPORAL EXPECTATIONS

In undertaking academic learning and research, everyone combines different rhythms of time. We exist in all modes of times that ripple out all at once, through which we must search for ways to accomplish our goals and academic demands. Current organisational policies, study and work conditions in the higher education sector significantly impact the mental health of university students (Levecque et al., 2017). We can experience constant strain due to the time and energy consuming practices that keep pushing us into an unhealthy work-life style. The meaning of 'full participation' is assumed as a complex entanglement of intensities, dimensions, timeframes, and speeds (Vandenbussche & De Schauwer, 2017). Ableism and excellence are idealised and valued highly. Being included means paradoxically complying with temporal progression and engagement (Whitburn & Thomas, 2021). It is relevant to all (PHD) students that we can look critically to these neoliberal framing of time in universities.

A possible danger of this meaning of time is that universities pose disabling contexts for (doctoral) students, with little room for difference (Brown, 2021). Yet, in a hyper-productive environment, our experiences with being short-in-time can be intensified by the demands of life. For example, time is differentially measurable for people with disabilities. Normative time frames need to be approached flexible than, and this flow can be unsustainable in the longer term: strategies over a protracted period create time bombs as the additional efforts are not endless. Basing on my own experiences as a (doctoral) student who is vision impaired, I will show how I encountered temporal barriers. In describing examples of how I am differentially temporal, I try to crip time in academia. Like Alison Kafer (2013) states:

> Crip time is flex time not just expanded but exploded; it requires re-imagining our notions of what can and should happen in time, or recognizing how expectations of 'how long things take' are based on very particular minds and bodies. Rather than bend disabled bodies and minds to meet the clock, crip time bends the clock to meet disabled bodies and minds.

At the same time, we can also encounter other notions of time in academia, specifically, those found in the disciplines of disability studies and (post)qualitative research inquiries. Understanding this time is formed through the interrelatedness of taking time, occurring in time, and time through reflection and depth (Chi Wing Lau, 2019; Titchkosky, 2010). It is about finding a slower form of scholarly being, a different type of productivity. Relationally being in it together whereby time is doing something in the process. It is finding "more time to think, to digest, and even to misunderstand each other in building a dialogue between the natural sciences and humanities" (Bozalek, 2017, p. 45). It is standing still, or seeing slowly, that reveals what might otherwise be quick to overlook (Ulmer, 2016). Reciprocity and slowness are of high importance to make space for contextualization and complexity. By circling and re-circling, conceptualizing and re-conceptualizing, searching and re-searching/researching; the strict temporal procedures that pose limitations and ableism can be disturbed and overruled, in favour of a human, collective, circular sense of time.

This chapter is about struggling with time, experiencing academic time pressures, needing more time to do things or using time differently when you live with a disability. Placing my experiences as a doctoral student directly in the field of vision, is setting the time to watch the synchronising of different temporalities. I incorporate a complexity of multiple contradictory rhythms and workings of time where several speeds continually crisscross. I take time to fulfil necessary engagements. I search for other modes of time, providing small cracks, or cripping time. Students with disabilities have the power to time travel, creating new rhythms of time and attuning their inner clock to the system.

DISABILITY AS AN INTENSIFIER

Disability and time are inextricably linked with each other. Living with a disability can be experienced as a time-intensive process and implies the complexity of juggling additional time-consuming activities. Dominant temporal regimes and schedules that encourage particular rhythms, paces and work scales, do not align with disability (Chi Wing Lau, 2019). In the bureaucratic structures and framing of time by universities, disability is taken for granted in a problematic and avoidable way. As a result, the academic journey of disabled students is frequently affected: additional efforts and extra workload shrink our time. We are structurally subjected to pressures; we must overcompensate for our disability in these temporal regimes, and we must acknowledge these efforts. Yet, the clock does not slow down because we need more time.

Living with a vision impairment creates particular challenges comprising additional roles (Jammaers & Williams, 2021). For instance, I must find time to undertake hospital appointments and rehabilitation sessions. Medical (eye care) consultations, mobility lessons and those for activities of daily living, and disability-specific follow-up conversations also take place during working hours and at locations outside the office, which all involve additional time. Exploring the environment, housing "alone", building and sustaining (new) social networks, and organizing shopping of daily living are other activities related to living away from a familiar home and near a university. On the one hand, I need to perform necessary and conditional time-consuming actions because of my impairment (Bulk, 2020). On the other hand, my tempo is personally experienced slower or not compatible with my impression of the expected rhythm of fellows (Brown, 2021; Whitburn & Thomas, 2021). I must do more in less time which provides pressures, and the complex balancing act of self-care and (over)compensation takes up much of my time.

Perpetuating ableism in academia and intern pushing thoughts conflict with my need to slow down, being forced to choose slowness over speed and rethinking daily life, due to the impairment of fostering a long-term, healthy, sustainable, balanced, and meaningful way of being. The amount of work is not adapted to what can get done in the productive hours. It feels more like a balancing act between utilising pre-identified adjustments and still failing to comply with the normative timeframes of academic culture of speed. This, quite simply, needs to change. Students with disabilities can explore their time, incorporating all intensities. Rethinking normativity, independence, and autonomy in how we are using time is helpful not only for students with disabilities, but for all people involved at university. Students with disabilities can help to put this on the table.

PREPARATION AND CONCENTRATION

Undertaking a similar level of intellectual engagement and fulfilling tasks equal to colleagues often requires greater time investment on my part. In relation to undertaking readings and writing a thesis or assessment work, certain actions require additional time, concentration, and collaboration. For example, I must invest longer periods of time reading relevant literature using a screen reader. Developing artisan skills and collaborating with support is also necessary in the analysis stage of a study, due to the inability/inaccessibility of relevant software. External assistance is invariably needed to support referencing and formatting, and other visual support is needed to lay out presentations. In these cases, I must first prepare the content, after which to negotiate with my personal assistant until we reach an acceptable result, which is accessible to me and visually attractive for audience. Schematising substantial amounts of data also demands extra-temporal engagement. All of this not only asks for intense additional efforts; it also leads to physical and emotional exhaustion.

It is not difficult to understand how the above can impact on my concentration levels, and those of other students with disabilities. Working harder, for longer hours, is challenging. To craft a balance for myself, I attempt to control the length of days by working part-time at a daily average of six hours. But my study/employment circumstances often demand more work hours, forcing me to adjust to the needs of the educational/research program. While it may be possible on an individual basis to discuss progress and build in flexibility with supervisors, this is not always possible nor aligned with the structured milestones and ultimate expectations of an academic program. Customising the trajectory is difficult because essential tasks are often neither adjustable nor redistributable. The institutional and governmental rights and underlying laws need to become negotiable in favour of inspirational and differential practices.

Disability also demands extra time for daily living. Functioning in an able-bodied study/work environment involves the need for pre-planning and it can require additional energy. For example, customising things with braille labels or memorizing workarounds of the microwave and coffee machine. Help from others (or in other words, their time) still stays necessary. Additional external audits, communication with IT managers, drawing an alliance with another impaired person of the university, the installation of extra software, … have all been necessary to enable functioning. I even find myself needing to "educate" the cleaning team, asking if they could return the dustbins to the same place every time they clean, and not to place chairs on the tables with the legs upwards. This is a form of self-advocacy, which is yet another demand on personal time. The design of the institution can be a constraint. Even flexible workplaces and open offices can be unworkable due to the sensory overstimulation and constant variability of the environment. Finding your way around such an environment can present ongoing hindrances.

Collaborating with a diverse group of colleagues is already potentially fraught. With a disability, this can be magnified, and requires an attentive attitude and the time for negotiation. For vision impaired people, for example, it is difficult to recognise others, or pick-up on non-verbal communication in group conversations; a lot of (in)formal exchanges and photos might be missed. It feels awkward to have social conversations not knowing who you are speaking to or participating in meetings when you do not know who is there. Compensating in such events often needs extra efforts. I sometimes miss on the "fun" moments, taking recuperation time due to fatigue because of impairment effects, which fellows or the university administration are unaware is happening. The functioning of everyone must be collectively supported, which requires a rethinking of how we "do" time together.

ACCESSIBILITY OF THE WORK ENVIRONMENT

Persons with a disability can request reasonable adjustments in the level of organisation, content, proportions, circumstances, and conditions of their engagement. However, this aspect of the support system is often individualized and time consuming to navigate. In the university, I need to learn how the "reasonable adjustments" system works and spent many hours following up on almost every aspect. The onus falls on the student—I am expected to take responsibility for my support needs in the process. While this appears logical, it is often experienced as an inefficiency. A student with a disability cannot start making arrangements to enable disability-specific support before their first day, for reasons that in some cases it may not be clear what sort of support they might need. As a result, the starting period of administrative formalities is time-consuming, and delays are almost always inevitable. At my institution, it was impossible to officially employ a personal assistant for a project application writing process, and it took more than six months until she could begin to provide me the necessary support.

Accessibility standards are now included in many areas of higher education institutions (Titchkosky, 2010). But accessibility requirements are implicated in our temporal capacity to study, which can challenge and shrink our time to focus on actual work. For the student with a vision impairment, for example, printed textbooks or course materials need to be scanned by hand or obtained electronically, which requires external help and additional time. Existing digital documents are not always automatically readable, and these need to be remediated or retrofitted to provide accessibility. The internet, digital classrooms (or Learning Management Systems), and library platforms with publications are often not designed with universal design principles. Searching or reading information online is, as a result, an overwhelming and excessively time-consuming task. Paradoxically, I ask my personal assistant to explore the literature and to send accessible versions of resources, instead of learning to work around or deal differently with these challenges. While it is time-consuming to communicate with someone else, it is more efficient than struggling repeatedly on my own with time bearing down. It would be time saving if accessible access to all materials existed for everyone.

Mobility is also often taxing on time for disabled people. People who are vision impaired, for example, are highly dependent on public transport or taxis. But walking and using public transport to reach the campus is a highly concentrated exercise. Safety and fluidity of moving might be challenged because of route changes or road works. An occupational therapist trained me to use a cane, and to be attentive to landmarks. Orientation and mobility sessions are intensive, and each route requires repetition. Familiar routes become a habit but moving for me is never an opportunity to relax. I am constantly forward planning: "Next traffic Island is the bus stop; pay attention to the cyclists on your left; two meters after the traffic sign is the pedestrian crossing." Locational crafting by using the ability of telework can cut down the hours needed to reach the department. Searching or understanding visual prompts or applying GPS guidance takes more time and the safety of the roads cannot be estimated. To collect research data at participants' homes, or attending conferences, is additionally challenging because of physical issues. The schedule of the university does not typically account for these temporal engagements in its temporal design.

RECOMMENDATIONS FOR INSTITUTIONAL IMPROVEMENT

I belong in academia, as does every disabled person. But the inaccessibility of time related resources and facilities raises important questions. My experiences in academia as a vision impaired person challenge the stereotype of disability in able-bodied culture and includes the embodiment of temporarily corporeal difference in the conversation. My experiences are not particularly unique in academia. Time weighs on all of us. Institutions need to re-structure academic temporality in traditional paths: reclaiming time for learning and doing research, being able to prioritise reading, thinking, and writing about the topic (Chi Wing Lau, 2019). Temporal differentiation (Whitburn & Thomas, 2021) could enable people to balance their jobs, additional tasks, and personal time engagements. This is not solely of high significance or relevance for disabled people, but for everyone who experiences time pressures in their work as a (doctoral) student, often in combination with personal and family live. The issue, for everyone, is to scale the value of the intensifier(s) in the workload in a healthier way that respects the extra efforts and takes away unnecessary barriers.

The current flow of academic time is a barrier to inclusion. Academic institutions can slow things down. Developing knowledge cannot be a linear path and cannot follow the traditional rhythms of the clock. This chapter calls for a de-escalation and slowing of the pace and volume of academic production and performativity, not only for disabled students, but for all scholars. It challenges the institution to de-prioritize speed, efficiency, acceleration, output, and standardized timelines in academic work.

We need to talk about time, and how the institutional concept of time continues to confront students with a disability with disablement and ableism in this very privileged environment. Students who live with disabilities should be able to work at their own pace. Each expression of struggling with or fighting the academic temporalities are meaningful small cracks that questions or moves the institutional system and its attitudes.

Such a rethinking of academic time is a collective action. Sharing experiences of contradictory temporalities makes everyone aware of what happens or needs to happen, as a meaningfully form of education. An individual fighting the system does not work. This asks for slow learning together; it asks for coalitions. We need to try alternatives, grow our small cracks upwards, as well as disrupt and resist the existing model of institutional time. We need to imagine different ways of being and becoming in time: cripping time, by exploring creative and flexible temporalities.

REFERENCES

Bozalek, V. (2017). Slow scholarship in writing retreats: A diffractive methodology for response-able pedagogies. *South African Journal of Higher Education, 31*(2), 40–57.

Brown, N. (Ed.). (2021). *Lived experiences of ableism in academia. Strategies for inclusion in higher education*. Policy Press.

Bulk, L. Y. (2020). *Being blind and belonging in academia* [Unpublished doctoral dissertation]. University of British Columbia. https://doi.library.ubc.ca/10.14288/1.0395453

Chi Wing Lau, T. (2019). Slowness, disability, and academic productivity: The need to rethink academic culture. In C. McMaster & B. Whitburn (Eds.), *Disability and the university: A disabled students' manifesto* (pp. 11–19). Peter Lang.

Jammaers, E., & Williams, J. (2021). Care for the self, overcompensation and bodily crafting: The work–life balance of disabled people. *Gender, Work & Organization, 28*(1), 119–137. https://doi.org/10.1111/gwao.12531

Kafer, A. (2013). *Feminist queer crip*. Bloomington: Indiana University Press.

Levecque, K., Anseel, F., De Beuckelaer, A., Van der Heyden, J., & Gisle, L. (2017). Work organization and mental health problems in PhD students. *Research Policy, 46*(4), 868–879. https://doi.org/10.1016/j.respol.2017.02.008

Titchkosky, T. (2010). The not-yet time of disability in the bureaucratization of university life. *Disability Studies Quarterly, 30*(3/4). http://www.dsq-sds.org/article/view/1295/1331

Ulmer, J. B. (2016). Writing slow ontology. *Qualitative Inquiry*. https://doi.org/10.1177/1077800416643994

Vandenbussche, H., & De Schauwer, E. (2017). The pursuit of belonging in inclusive education—insider perspectives on the meshwork of participation. *International Journal of Inclusive Education*, *22*(9), 969–982. https://doi.org/10.1080/13603116.2017.1413686

Whitburn, B., & Thomas, M. K. E. (2021). A right to be included: The best and worst of times for learners with disabilities. *Scandinavian Journal of Disability Research*, *23*(1), 104–113. https://doi.org/10.16993/sjdr.772

CHAPTER 3

Slowness, Disability, and Academic Productivity: The Need to Rethink Academic Culture

TRAVIS CHI WING LAU

INTRODUCTION

The increasing corporatization of higher education in America and in many other countries has perpetuated a long-standing academic culture of hyper-productivity—one that privileges speed, efficiency, and results. Colloquially referred to as "publish or perish," this prevailing model of academic work depends on an increasingly untenable set of metrics to determine a scholars' contribution to their respective fields and institutions. Scholars who fail to publish enough peer-reviewed articles or monographs while simultaneously teaching their required course loads (up to three to four classes per quarter or semester) and serving on numerous academic and administrative committees frequently risk having tenure delayed or even denied entirely. Instructors are tasked with larger and larger class sizes and higher enrollment caps, while being expected to be available to their students as much as possible. Early-career academics and an expanding population of adjunct laborers bear the brunt of mounting demands for productivity and increased scrutiny, both at departmental and institutional levels. In the face of fewer and fewer tenure-track positions and deepening departmental budget cuts, graduate programs have reinforced this ethos of speed through both the structures of graduate study and their strategies for professionalization. The "crisis" rhetoric dominating discourses about the current state of the humanities has, rather than sounding a call to action, unfortunately only served to intensify and normalize pressure to comply with the demands of academic productivity. Overwork, constant work, and fast work are not only the new normal; they are framed as necessary in the face of dire circumstances.

In this chapter, I consider how disabled scholars are actively excluded by the dominant temporal regimes of the neoliberal university. How does the academy inculcate certain modes of productivity and at what costs? How does the academic culture of speed, in its desire for persistent and consistent output, actually disable its very laborers and stifle the work that they do? The nature of quality academic scholarship—as a series of extended acts of thinking, reading, writing, and editing—is antithetical to the current rhythms (or perhaps arrhythmia) of contemporary academic life. By drawing together critiques of normative time and theories of "crip time" posed by disability studies with recent discussions of "slow scholarship," this chapter makes a case for resisting the culture of speed in favor of more accessible and sustainable models of academic labor that better serve both scholars and their scholarship.

THE ACADEMIC CULTURE OF SPEED

One of the primary means by which academics are indoctrinated into the culture of speed is through their graduate training. Graduate programs not only provide necessary introductions to the fundamentals of a field, but also socialize young scholars into the norms of their profession. As more students attend graduate school immediately upon completion of their undergraduate studies, graduate programs often serve as formative spaces for those students to transition into their identities as scholars-in-training and as academic laborers who provide services to their institutions. New graduate students are often required to enroll in 3–4 seminars per semester and, depending on scheduling, may attend within the same day multiple class sessions that meet for 2–3 hours. Dwindling departmental funding for students beyond their fifth or sixth years also compels many graduate students to take as many courses as possible in their first and second years of study in order to finish on time. Many institutions also expect graduate students to teach undergraduate courses that require extensive preparation.

The pace of seminars frequently leads to compressed periods of overwork during a typical fifteen-week semester. Alongside multiple in-class presentations, students are expected to keep up with reading loads that sometimes amount to multiple full academic monographs each week. This reading is frequently assigned all the way to the final week of the semester, which then forces students to either prioritize researching and writing their own final projects (which represents most, if not all, of their grade) or the assigned material for class. While it is fair to say that graduate school encourages students to learn strategies for time management to prevent the overwork I am describing, the demands of having four classes with overlapping deadlines make slow, distributed work immensely difficult, if not impossible. Many of my graduate-student colleagues have resorted to judicious selection of seminar readings or even hierarchizing their seminars in terms of preparation or attendance. This kind of decision-making out of necessity has become *de rigueur* and runs entirely counter to the department's mission of exposing students to different historical periods, critical objects, or theoretical apparatuses. Students instead pick courses whose topics seem most useful to them or whose instructor may be a future committee member for an exam or dissertation. The exigencies of the seminar system preclude exploration, rereading, and contemplation, all of which might otherwise enrich a student's existing investment in a particular field or incite new interest in an entirely unfamiliar one. The closing down of possibility—at the moment when young graduate students most need room to grow—seems to be a missed opportunity in developing more well-rounded scholars early in their intellectual formation. While some institutions are beginning to reduce the number of courses required to fulfill doctoral requirements, the pacing and structure of these seminars still offer little time for students to slowly and thoroughly complete readings and written work.

Concluding seminar papers remain the privileged form of summative assessment in most graduate classrooms. While some professors are open to presentations that culminate in a final paper or other useful scholarly form of writing—such as the conference paper or the annotated bibliography—most prefer the traditional seminar paper of roughly 15–30 typed pages. Many first-year doctoral students in my department find themselves with upwards of 80 pages of writing to complete in the form of 4 entirely different research projects that are to be "of publishable quality." Often compressed within the last weeks of the semester, these papers seldom reach a level of "publishable" polish. Many graduate students, especially those without previous graduate experience, find themselves needing to request extensions or in some cases incomplete course status, which then puts their academic standings and wellbeing in jeopardy. These deferred, incomplete assignments sometimes carry over into subsequent semesters, effectively trapping students in a loop of incompleteness that impedes their progress in an already compressed degree timeline.

The expectation of "publishable" work at the seminar level is deeply ironic, given that the actual labor of producing publishable quality scholarship in the profession involves a prolonged process that rarely takes less than a year—many submissions require significant revision, guided by a lengthy peer review process, before resubmission and final publication (Hayot, 2014). What practical skills, then, do seminar papers actually offer graduate students, when they will never be asked to produce that amount of writing within such a narrow timeframe? What more do they teach than writing quickly under duress? This disconnect between professional reality and the seminar paper reveals just how unnecessary and misrepresentative these kinds of academic hurdles really are. Given that a surprising number of seminar papers receive little to no feedback aside from a grade, the seminar paper becomes counterproductive by demanding significant labor from graduate students, with an uncertain payoff aside from a requirement checked off their list. Very few students revisit these early seminar papers, a process which takes away valuable time and energy from teaching and dissertation writing, or do so much later in their careers when they can afford to substantially revise them into articles.

In extreme cases, I witnessed students ignoring course material outright to devote their semesters to producing would-be articles for publication, a choice which defeats the purpose of coursework and only furthers the competitive pressures within cohorts and in the greater academic community to "publish or perish." Some programs have begun to experiment with different course requirements, like having only one major paper due per semester or a lengthy reading period after the end of the course, but these measures fail to consider whether the seminar paper is a valuable measure of graduate student competency and progress at all. Instead of teaching graduate students writing methodologies or approaches to producing article-length or chapter-length pieces of writing, seminar papers only serve to perpetuate the pervasive anxiety of needing to publish and to do so quickly that follows young scholars into their early careers.

Course work and seminar requirements exemplify how speed and efficiency are valorized with regard to graduate student success. Comprehensive examinations are another example of a form of summative assessment that seems to be more about student endurance than their actual capacities to synthesize and reflect on the material they have studied. Varying across disciplines, these examinations are typically timed and involve oral components that require students to defend their exam responses or even demonstrate knowledge on the spot. Months of preparation may be condensed into a single day of examination. This expectation of quick thinking is usually justified as a necessity because scholars are expected to respond to questions posed to them after conference presentations or during job interviews. The exam is meant to help graduate students "practice" this skill.

Neuroatypical students or chronically ill/disabled students, many of whom may not be able to work within the temporal restrictions of exams, are set up to either fail or to request accommodations. In many cases, these requests are denied by the committee or the department on the basis of fairness. In my own experience, the chronic pain and accompanying brain fog caused by my scoliosis became a significant barrier to my completing an exam within 24 hours. Referred to informally by graduate students as a departmental hazing ritual, this exam encourages speedy reaction rather than slow production of robust responses to key questions and concepts relevant to a future dissertation project. Without advanced knowledge of the questions, there was simply too little time to plan and outline what needed to be essays of seminar paper length. The format of the exam forced me to work in spite of my disability, to the detriment of my wellbeing. The place of cognitive or intellectual disability (in my case, brain fog) "represents the near unthinkable of academia," which begs the question of whether or not the academic culture of speed leaves any space for neurodiversity (Chen, 2015, p. 177).

Cognitive differences, like brain fog, mark the limit cases for what kinds of bodyminds can exist in academia (Chen, 2015). What purports to be "rigor" in departmental justifications for such examinations is actually a deeply ableist system of values which forces graduate students to demonstrate their ability, as in the case of the seminar paper, to produce a form of academic writing that they will never be asked again in their professional careers to produce under the same conditions. These breathless forms of examination belie how "academic institutions we inhabit are at this moment adept at producing ... disciplined cognators," those who are able to display a particular kind of "thinking on your feet" cognitive style that processes and reacts quickly (Chen, 2015, p. 178). These "unhealthy forms of intellectual conformity" harm both the graduate students that develop the strategies and coping mechanisms to maintain this style of cognition and those that fail to comply at all (Kudlick, 2006, pp. 164–165). What are programs really teaching graduate students by suggesting that being "too slow" is failure?

Rather than actively excluding those who may not be capable of adapting to this form of cognition, departments need to recognize the implicit disciplining that is built into graduate training. Rigorous examinations need not be punitive to encourage preparation and strong performance; rather, they can demand the same level of intellectual engagement while allowing students to invest the time necessary to develop their lines of argumentation or, more practically, conceptualize a dissertation project. Alternative structures that accommodate longer periods of thinking and writing or shorter forms of writing would do better justice to student learning. How might the exam being reimagined to either allow for more space and time for play with ideas or to feed more directly into the writing of the dissertation proposal and a first chapter? Consider, for example, a "conference panel" format in which students present brief arguments and conclusions drawn from their reading and engage in dialogue with one another and their examiners. This collective knowledge-making exercise, rather than an exam for exam's sake, enables students to learn from one another, especially if they work in different fields.

Both of the examples I have chosen demonstrate how a culture of speed individualizes failure as a student's own inability to do good work. The prevalence of "imposter syndrome" among graduate students only underscores how pernicious this model of academic productivity and success can be, because it shifts attention away from the greater structural problems of the program itself toward the student as the obstacle to her own success (Brems et al., 1994; Clance & Imes, 1978; Harvey & Katz, 1984). Students frequently internalize the struggle to "keep up" in fear of being seen as less capable or unfit for the profession by mentors or peers. Because the tempo of graduate programs remains so fast, opportunities for self-care and separation from academic life become increasingly impossible. Most time-management advice manuals and graduate school primers tend to reinforce scheduled and highly organized time as a solution for the labor anxieties generated within the academic culture of speed (Berg & Seeber, 2016). By placing the burden back on the student to figure out a system that best enables them to maximize their own productivity, these texts leave unquestioned the ways in which present academic labor is structured to prevent good scholarship that may require its own forms of time. Scholarly ingenuity is less about actual innovative scholarship than about how the graduate student overcomes or outsmarts the ableist demands of academic life.

Graduate students and faculty need to work more closely together in the structuring of graduate programs that best train students in the actual skills of the profession, while recognizing and accommodating different forms of cognitive ability. That most programs have only one structure or path that all incoming students undergo suggests a lack of imagination in the ways graduate programs can better serve their diverse student bodies. The standardization of a graduate program across all cohorts presupposes a monolithic vision of scholars as identical thinkers, workers, and writers when that is simply not the case. We must work to enable the collective flourishing of scholars in body and mind rather than punish those who may not be able to comply. Graduate programs should not be disabling scholars and their scholarship.

CRIP AND SLOW

Crip time attends to how disability remains in tension with the dictates of normative time frames (Kafer, 2013; Kuppers, 2014; Price, 2011; Samuels, 2017). Crip time recognizes how disabled embodiment does not always align with work schedules and deadlines that encourage particular paces, rhythms, and scales of work: "Crip time refuses to define itself in terms of either the ideal or the average: Schedules for work, parenting, and the social are thus shaped by individual needs, desires, and abilities, rather than by regimented economic and cultural imperatives," (Samuels, 2006, p. 5). As a resistant orientation, crip time is necessarily *slow* because it is inflected by liminal states of disability and debility that refuse the fantasies of normalcy and regimented productivity. Many academic institutions have taken up crip time as another way of signaling later start times for events or the need for additional time for completing assignments or exams.

But this is a gross oversimplification of crip time that misses its potential to reorient our relationship, as scholars, to academic time:

> Crip time is flex time not just expanded but exploded; it requires reimagining our notions of what can and should happen in time, or recognizing how expectations of "how long things take" are based on very particular minds and bodies. We can then understand the flexibility of crip time as being not only an accommodation to those who need "more" time but also, and perhaps especially, a challenge to normative and normalizing expectations of pace and scheduling. Rather than bend disabled bodies and minds to meet the clock, crip time bends the clock to meet disabled bodies and minds. (Kafer, 2013, p. 27)

Academic labor might be better understood not as the quantifiable results of pages written, pieces published, or courses taught, but in terms of the psychic and physical labor that attends researching, writing, and thinking. This attention to the micro-level of disability experience, or what Merri Lisa Johnson has described as a "matter of intensities, sensations and situations," shifts the accommodation discussion away from reductive arguments about scarcity (i.e., "We simply can't accommodate everyone because we have too little resources of time and money!") toward reimagining an academic culture that different bodies relate with time differently (2014, p. 135). Rather than having scholars work at the mercy of strict academic clocks, we can bend those clocks to meet disabled bodies where they are. This explosion of normative modalities of time (hyper-productivity, efficiency, constant progress) also explodes our narrow visions of an academic future "deployed in the service of compulsory able-bodiedness and able-mindedness" (Kafer, 2013, p. 27). At the rate and manner we are working, we are projecting an academic future that does not have disabled scholars in it.

"Slow scholarship" or "slow academia" is a nascent academic movement that has asked urgent questions about the material consequences for scholars working within an increasingly breathless academic culture of speed under neoliberal university governance. Taking inspiration from the Slow Food movement, and the more recent "Slow Science Manifesto" (2010), Berg and Seeber's *The Slow Professor: Challenging the Culture of Speed in the Academy* lays out a similar manifesto for moving toward a culture of slow scholarship in the humanities:

> Slow Professors advocate deliberation over acceleration. We need time to think, and so do our students. Time for reflection and open-ended inquiry is not a luxury but is crucial to what we do ... We envisage Slow Professor acting purposefully, cultivating emotional and intellectual resilience. By taking the time for reflection and dialogue, the Slow Professor takes back the intellectual life the university. (2016, p. x)

Disability concepts like crip time offer complementary conceptual models of academic temporality. Rather than simply "reclaiming" time for thinking and writing or refusing time-consuming tasks like email, a "crip slow" approach pushes us to be more critical of larger structures of productivity that are tied to academic progression like publication and graduate training. Both professors *and* students have something to gain from a "crip slow" approach that recognizes how rigid structures of academic labor work to disable both populations, especially as faculty reproduce microcosms of this larger culture within classrooms and departments.

The invisible forms of labor that disabled students and faculty have done to navigate the current culture of academic speed needs to be recognized *as labor* so that we might begin to imagine structures that do not constrain the work of good scholarship. This might begin with a revision of hiring criteria, and even tenure requirements, that tend to overemphasize the number of peer-reviewed articles and monographs published as proof of scholarly productivity. Given that achieving tenure remains a primary goal for many early-career academics, departments have a responsibility to consider the consequences of these metrics and the accelerated timelines they encourage and enforce. The "ailing" job market is no excuse for cultivating an academic culture that actively excludes scholars whose labor may not be legible in the same ways. What gets to count as "productivity" demands much more scrutiny than those who may fail to be "productive."

Critics of "slow scholarship" dismiss the movement as a privileged idealism for those more established in their careers, those who can afford to be "slow" in the first place. Instead of reproducing the division between tenured and non-tenured faculty, "slow scholarship" might instead find solidarity with anti-casualization movements that aim to protect contingent laborers like adjuncts whose labor continues to be undervalued in the academy (Lopes & Dewan, 2015; Standing, 2011). By recognizing how scholars at every stage of their careers can enable the work of others in the academy by making time and space for them, "slow scholarship" is a *collective* project to remake the university with an ethics of care and interdependence rather than simply "slow scholarship" done on the backs of the academic precariat (Mountz et al., 2015). Academic freedom should not involve only the right to free inquiry, but also the right of different bodyminds to do that scholarship in a sustainable work culture that does not thrive at the expense of their wellbeing.

REFERENCES

Berg, M., & Seeber, B. K. (2016). *The slow professor: Challenging the culture of speed in the academy.* Toronto, Canada: University of Toronto Press.

Brems, C., Baldwin, M. R., Davis, L., & Namyniuk, L. (1994). The imposter syndrome as related to teaching evaluations and advising relationships of university faculty members. *Journal of Higher Education, 65*(2), 183–193.

Chen, M. Y. (2015). Brain fog: The race for cripistemology. *Journal of Literary & Cultural Disability Studies, 8*(2), 171–184.

Clance, P. R., & Imes, S. (1978). The imposter phenomenon in high achieving women: Dynamics and therapeutic intervention. *Psychotherapy Theory, Research and Practice, 15*(3), 241–247.

Harvey, J. C., & Katz, C. (1984). *If I'm so successful, why do I feel like a fake?* New York, NY: Random House.

Hayot, E. (2014). *The elements of academic style: Writing for the humanities.* New York, NY: Columbia University Press.

Kafer, A. (2013). *Feminist, queer, crip.* Bloomington, IN: Indiana University Press.

Kudlick, C. (2006). A history profession for everybody. *Journal of Women's History, 18*(1), 163–167.

Kuppers, P. (2014). Crip time. *Tikkun Magazine, 29*(4), 29–31.

Lopes, A., & Dewan, I. (2015). Precarious pedagogies? The impact of casual and zero-hour contracts in higher education. *Journal of Feminist Scholarship, 7*(8), 28–42.

Mountz, A., Bonds, A., Mansfield, B., Loyd, J., Hyndman, J., Walton-Roberts, M., ... Curran, W. (2015). For slow scholarship: A feminist politics of resistance through collective action in the neoliberal university. *ACME: An International Journal for Critical Geographies, 14*(4), 1235–1259.

Price, M. (2011). *Mad at school: Rhetorics of mental disability and academic life.* Ann Arbor, MI: University of Michigan Press, 2011.

Samuels, E. (2006, January). *Normative time: How queerness, disability, and parenthood impact academic labor.* Paper presented at the Modern Language Association Annual Meeting, Philidelphia, PA.

Samuels, E. (2017). Six ways of looking at crip time. *Disability Studies Quarterly, 37*(3). Retrieved from: http://dx.doi.org/10.18061/dsq.v37i3.5824

Standing, G. (2011). *The precariat: The new dangerous class.* New York, NY: Bloomsbury Academic.

CHAPTER 4

Disability Advocacy Within the Ableist Environment of Academia

DENISE BECKWITH

INTRODUCTION: "NOTHING ABOUT ME WITHOUT ME"

Disability advocacy is a means of overcoming academic ableism. Educational participation is a human right, one that should not be withheld from people with disabilities. People have often wondered why I have chosen to remain at a university where I have encountered ableism and discrimination, needing to undertake disability advocacy not only for myself but for the benefit of other students and staff with disabilities. Ableism occurs in all sections of the community. Tertiary education is no exception as it, too, is reflective of a bureaucracy that is ableist in nature. I remain in academia because people with disabilities need to be present and visible to bring about change in higher education.

I have a physical impairment; I use crutches for mobility. At university I receive participatory support in the form of a practical assistant who is appointed to assist me with physical tasks associated with undertaking high degree research, inclusive of typing, presentation preparation and research assistance. I returned to study at an Australian university having worked in the disability advocacy sector for 16 years. I wanted to undertake a degree that was relevant to both my work and lived-experience. I decided to undertake a Bachelor of Social Work with the intention of progressing to a PhD, naively believing that there would be an understanding of structural disadvantage that comes with disability and that I would not need to provide detailed explanations of my particular requirements. This belief stemmed from the understanding that social work and social sciences, as disciplines relevant to social interaction, would be more socially aware. There was an expectation that academics, as tertiary education is equated with the best and brightest, would be more open-minded to forms of difference such as disability, and would understand it as only an element of identity. Unfortunately, this was not reflected. Constant justification and explanation of disability was a necessity.

In this chapter I highlight experiences as an undergraduate, postgraduate and an academic that will guide and advise students with disability in university settings so tertiary institutions can learn from lived-experience to ensure mistakes are not repeated. This chapter will explain how to use advocacy and consultation to address inequity and inaccessibility within academia to ensure it is more inclusive and reflective of wider society.

"WHY DO YOU NEED THAT?": EXPLANATION SYNDROME

I am based at a university which provides disability support to students who request it or to those who disclose having a disability and require reasonable adjustments. This ableist approach puts the onus on the individual to disclose details about their disability in order to have their individual needs met. This has the potential to cause people with disability to see their disability as a barrier instead of an asset to the development of their knowledge (Dolmage, 2017).

Throughout my academic career, inclusive of my current PhD study, there has been a continual expectation that I provide justification and explanation for disability adjustments before anything will be provided to me. This has involved the provision of medical evidence, which in its own right is a form of ableism as it calls upon the professional expertise a medical professional rather than relying on the person's lived-experience and knowledge. Ableism is using medical evidence to "other" and separate those who are non-normative due to disability and bodily difference (Campbell, 2009). This contravenes the social definition of disability—that there are environmental and attitudinal barriers that cause discrimination and inequity (Mitra, 2018)

It is an expectation that PhD students attend academic conferences to expand their professional networks and disseminate information about their respective research in order to promote not only themselves but also their educational institution. But participatory assistance requirements increase the financial outlay of the university (Dolmage, 2017). I have had to debate the relevance, the reasons why, and the benefits of attending conferences for both myself and the university. The university bureaucracy makes a distinction between the types of assistance it will provide, and this is only associated with the completion of tertiary study—referred to as practical assistance—and is not in any way personal care assistance, such as toileting, dressing or support with eating. My needs, the institution has argued, come under personal care and are not within the scope of the practical assistant position.

A justification has to sometimes be provided to people who work within the disability support service who, by implication, should understand and represent the needs of people with disabilities across the university—ensuring that it is inclusive of that population.

Do tertiary institutions want to have students with disabilities for statistical purposes and financial benefits?—Do they want to appear inclusive to potential students and donors? These financial and social benefits to the university do not automatically translate to access and inclusion for students with disability. Argument, justification and explanation have to be undertaken by the student. The onus is on the student with disability, and results in people with disabilities having to constantly employ self-advocacy skills. Ideally, this is a situation that should change.

Until then, however, students must learn to be effective advocates by being present, visible and engaged so it becomes apparent that they are assets and valid members of institutions. This can be through academic participation (expressing views within tutorials and lectures) and political participation (student representative councils and members of disability collectives) as there is power in numbers. Tertiary institutions should not only include students with disabilities in consultation processes but also showcase them in promotional materials, websites and academic activities so that disability is normalised and accepted as a valid identity.

"WE'RE GETTING THE HELL OUT OF HERE, YOU SORT YOURSELF OUT!": EMERGENCY RESPONSES TO DISABILITY

During a mid-semester tutorial, a fire emergency occurred which resulted in smoke alarms being activated. I was left in the tutorial room by the tutor as they facilitated the evacuation of the other students, including some with disabilities who happened to be mobile. As a person with a mobility impairment, I was left to my own devices, the only support available to me being my practical assistant. Even the fire warden, who was directing people down the main stairs to the outdoor emergency assembly point, directed my practical assistant to leave me alone. There was no indication about what I was meant to do except that I was to make my own way out. Fortunately, my practical assistant protested and refused to leave me.

The same incident occurred twice within the period of a fortnight and the response from the University was exactly the same. The tutor left the building taking those students who could move, and I was left once again with my practical assistant. I actually felt that my life was being treated in a eugenic way—I felt I was disposable or of less value than the other students. After these incidents, I arranged to have a consultation meeting with the disability advisor and other staff associated with work, health and safety responses.

Academic institutions need to ensure proper training is provided in relation to responding to the needs of people with disabilities. They also need to acknowledge that these students pay the same fees and are thus entitled to the same protective responses. Making a complaint can ensure that work health and safety training within the university will be inclusive of disability and provide education for faculty in relation to appropriate responses. Modifications can be made to buildings to ensure there are accessible emergency exits including doors, automated entry, and gradients of exit ramps. My self-advocacy has led to the changing of work, health and safety modules to ensure they reflect the specific requirements of people with disabilities during emergency evacuation processes.

Students should consider the nature of the support that they require in the case of an emergency. This is part of reasonable adjustment requirements and can include such things as being close to a door and ensuring that there are no obstructions that would impede entrance and exit points. Disability support services and security staff should be approached to develop a plan and work in collaboration with not only students with disabilities, but security staff and work, health and safety committees to ensure emergency responses are implemented. None of what is being suggested can be done in isolation; students should regard themselves as assets to the university rather than burdens, so do not be afraid of accessing services that are available to make the student experience as safe and inclusive as possible.

"INTO THE CRIP CORNER": INCLUSION, NOT INTEGRATION

Integration is the societal expectation that people with disabilities will simply fit in without society having to make adjustments. Integration has the potential of being forcible and divisive (Oliver, 2009). I prefer inclusion. Inclusion is adopting a collective approach and seeing the benefits people with disabilities can bring to the wider community (Oliver, 2009). In one class I attended with two other students who happened to also have a disability, we were assigned groups to undertake a tutorial activity. As students with disability, we were grouped as three. This may have been done for the sake of convenience and based upon physical proximity rather than ensuring diversity within groups. It was an example of integration—we were in the class, but not a real part of it. To allocate all the students with disabilities to one group potentially magnified disability as a negative attribute and something to be avoided. We were set aside as different, rather than university students just as our peers. This incident illustrates the importance of providing training for casual sessional tutors to ensure inclusive practices are understood and adhered to.

Universities need to acknowledge that students with disabilities are not defined by their condition. The actions of the tutor reflected a rhetoric of integration which brought about the expectation that people with disabilities who are students are fitted in to the class and not active and valuable participants. Academic institutions should regard students with disabilities as an asset, beneficial to schools of the university, academics and students. Exposure to disability is in itself educative, as it has the capacity to enhance people's understanding of the lived-experience of disability. This is essential as disability can then be seen as an element of identity with cultural aspects (Dunn et al., 2008; McRuer, 2006). Universities can be inclusive of disability by ensuring their curricula interweaves disability across content and research rather than a specialist tokenistic topic that students can undertake if they have an interest (Davis, 2015). Students with disability should contemplate sharing their lived-experience, stories and knowledge as these are, in effect, educational.

"TO EMPLOY OR NOT EMPLOY!": DISABILITY IN ACADEMIA

Universities need to be more conscious of inclusive employment policies as people with disability are under-represented in academic positions, reinforcing societal assumptions that we do not have the capacity to deliver lectures, teach, assess or undertake research. Ableist knowledge is the only knowledge that is deemed valuable by universities whereas they should encourage diversity that is reflective of the wider community. By adopting affirmative action policies when employing people with disability, universities can be environments that have the potential to bring about social change so academics with disabilities do not feel that they are alone and are a constant educative tool (Campbell, 2009). This will result in universities being truly reflective of the community. There are also student benefits to having academics with disabilities in the form of providing exposure and equipping them in relation to professional development.

Universities can be more inclusive by having events that foster pride and recognition of all students including students with disabilities. This could be done by having disability inclusion or diversity weeks that encompass and showcase disability as an asset.

Students with disability may want to join disability collective groups on university campuses and connect to social media groups.

"I AM NEVER GOING TO WORK WITH PEOPLE WITH DISABILITY": DISABILITY INCLUSION, EMPLOYMENT AND ATTITUDES

"I am not going to work with people with disability so I don't need to know about it." This has been said to me by students I have taught, people I have worked with, and students I have studied with, proving the statement ridiculous. It is a shocking and naive statement. 15% of the world's population has a disability making it the largest minority group globally (Shakespeare, 2017). It is a fallacy that disability can be avoided in a work context. This is especially so in the tertiary setting. What needs to be examined in each institution is how far disability services are equated with specialist services and expertise, when they should be about making the university accessible to and inclusive of everyone.

As an academic I have had students underestimate my ability to teach due to my disability. There is an expectation that I must justify what I know and how I know it. I had one student inform me that as they were intending to enter law enforcement they would not come into contact with people with disabilities. I highlighted to the student that people with disabilities also come in contact with police and the criminal justice system, as both victims and perpetrators, so they would knowingly or unknowingly come in contact with people with disabilities and have to respond to them (Hepner et al., 2015).

"DISABILITY IS NOT A DIRTY WORD": THE POWER OF LANGUAGE

There is a growing trend within academia to whitewash disability using alternative language such as "differently abled" or "diverse" in place of disability (Davis, 2015; O'Neill, 2011), attributable to a "politically correct" urge of not wanting to cause offence and due to perceived social stigma associated with the "d" word. This presents multiple risks, as disability is not seen as a structural and social disadvantage (Terzi, 2004). Another risk is students with disabilities internalizing the messages that normalcy, perfection and health are the only acceptable attributes within society and that disability equals deficiency and dysfunction (Campbell, 2009).

In one lecture I attended the lecturer was reluctant to show videos about disability in my presence, despite my preference that the educational resources be used and discussed, as able-bodied students could then see disability as a legitimate and significant topic.

One academic encouraged me to use "differently abled" as the descriptor for disability in my PhD research. What I walked away with was the feeling that non-disabled academics do not understand the politics of engagement within the disability community, a community that I do not get to leave as I am a person with disability. If I do not use the word disability I would be accused of being ableist. The greater proportion of the disability community do not use the term "differently abled" as they see disability as an identity and would argue that alternate terminology is used to make the non-disabled population more comfortable by emphasizing "ability," what Mairs referred to as a utopian philosophy (1986). A focus on equality for people with disability, rather than equity, ensures that people with disability are pushed to societal margins and not able to have a voice (McRuer, 2006).

Professors, lecturers and tutors need to lead by example and use the word disability or impairment as it is increasing students' understanding of the area of Disability Studies. Disability Studies is the acknowledgement that nobody wants to be in isolation and considered part of a minority. It is acknowledgement that people with disabilities cannot be considered as a homogenous group with a singular identity feature (Siebers, 2008). The use of the word disability by academic staff and students with disability illustrates that |Disability Studies and disability as an identity warrants exploration as disability is the largest minority group globally. The use of language associated with disability identity can contribute a great deal to the normalization of disability. Utilizing resources such as academic texts and materials that are inclusive of disability can also create normalization. Students with disabilities may want to consider leading by example and when responding to assessments across various areas of study, contemplate incorporating responses inclusive of disability so academics and fellow students can see that disability is a valuable area of study and should not be approached as an afterthought or specialist area.

"WHAT TOOK YOU SO LONG?": ACCESSIBILITY BEYOND THE MINIMUM

Building access codes are merely the minimum standards that should be addressed, they do not consider *individual* needs and requirements. It is a "ticking the box" response. Try walking to a campus that is being promoted as both accessible to, and inclusive of, students with disability. Invite people who have different roles within the planning of the campus. When I did this at a new campus, two of the party walked ahead of me, not aware of the amount of energy that I was expending. When we arrived at the campus they suggested that it was achievable. Yet a non-disabled walk of 850 meters, which should take about four minutes, took me 31 minutes in one direction and 40 minutes return.

Even when the surrounding environment is flat with numerous routes to walk, planners may not realise that "flatness" is not the only aspect of accessibility. Within the pathways on the walk there are subtle undulations and inclinations. A way to address this is to ensure campuses undertake access audits, these can be conducted by occupational therapists in consultation with students with disabilities. The benefit of access audits is they can be a learning opportunity for occupational therapy students as future professionals so they can practice skills associated with their profession.

To address access on university campuses, accessibility needs to be seen and interpreted in the broadest sense. For some people with disabilities, access equates to more than physical access. It can be inclusive of lighting design as lighting levels can exacerbate problems for people with vision or psychosocial impairment which can in turn impact upon functionality and productivity (Brawley, 2009).

"I HAVE SOMETHING TO SAY": ADVOCACY STRATEGIES

Advocacy is crucial for students with disabilities at universities. Advocacy brings about individual, systemic and sustained change. Within the bureaucratic structures of universities, allies are necessary. If critical issues are only to be discussed amongst the disability cohort/community there is a risk that nothing will change. Key to identifying allies is relationship and rapport building so that people move beyond seeing the master status of disability and see the whole person who is able to contribute to and participate in the university community—and beyond—in many different ways.

Advocacy can involve making complaints through both internal and external mechanisms. It is important to pursue complaints as it creates a precedent which results in structures being modified so current and future students with disabilities have an example and can use that to their advantage. It is important to come up with solutions using the professional language of the university because there are people who do not understand the subtleties and implications of disability. This is where lived-experience and clear communication is valuable. It takes student voices, action and identity pride to emphasize and promote student rights (Disability Advocacy Resource Unit, 2018). Universities have an obligation to consult students with disability to avoid making errors and to adhere to the philosophy of "nothing about us without us" (Charlton, 1998, p. 3). Student activism needs to include issues impacting upon people with disabilities and they need to have a position at the table or within consultation processes so that lived-experience and knowledge can be respected, acknowledged and learnt from.

REFERENCES

Brawley, E. (2009). Enriching lighting design. *Neuro Rehabilitation*, *25*(3), 189–199.
Campbell, F. K., (2009). *Contours of ableism: The production of disability and abledness*. London, UK: Palgrave Macmillan.
Charlton, J. I. (1998). *Nothing about us without us: Disability oppression and empowerment*. Berkley, CA: University of California Press.
Davis, L. J. (2015). Diversity. In R. Adams, B. Reiss, & D. Serlin (Eds.), *Keywords for disability studies* (Keywords series) (pp. 61–64). New York, NY: New York University Press.
Disability Advocacy Resource Unit. (2018). Retrieved from http://www.daru.org.au
Dolmage, J. T. (2017). *Academic ableism: Disability and higher education*. Ann Arbor, MI: University of Michigan Press.
Dunn, P., Hanes, R., Hardie, S., Leslie, D., & MacDonald, J. (2008). Best practices in promoting disability inclusion within Canadian schools of social work. *Disability Studies Quarterly*, *28*(1).
Hepner, I., Woodward, M. N., & Stewart, J. (2015). Giving the vulnerable a voice in the criminal justice system: The use of intermediaries with individuals with intellectual disability. *Psychiatry, Psychology and Law*, *22*(3), 453–464.
Mairs, N. (1986). *On being a cripple*. Retrieved from http://faculty.uml.edu/bmarshall/mairsonbeingacripple.pdf
McRuer, R. (2006). *Crip theory: Cultural signs of queerness and disability*. New York, NY: New York University Press.
Mitra, S. (2018). *Disability, health and human development* (Palgrave Studies in Disability and International Development). New York, NY: Palgrave Pivot.
Oliver, M. (2009). *Understanding disability: From theory to practice* (2nd ed.). Basingstoke, UK and New York: Palgrave Macmillan.
O'Neill, B. (2011). A critique of politically correct language (Essay). *Independent Review*, *16*(2), 279–291.
Shakespeare, T. (2017). *Disability: The basics*. London, UK: Routledge.
Siebers, T. (2008). *Disability theory* (Corporealities). Ann Arbor, MI: University of Michigan Press.
Terzi, L. (2004). The social model of disability: A philosophical critique. *Journal of Applied Philosophy*, *21*(2), 141–157.

CHAPTER 5

The Violent Consequences of Disclosure ... and How Disabled and Mad Students Are Pushing Back

FADY SHANOUDA

INTRODUCTION

Disclosing disability is a complicated and challenging process in higher education (Cheuk, 2012; Matthew, 2009; Kerschbaum et al., 2017). It includes submitting medical documentation, participating in assessments with disability service officers and medical experts, and arranging accommodations with professors and teaching assistants (Olney & Brockelman, 2003). Although disability service officers do conduct parts of the disclosure process in private, and students' medical information is legally protected in many countries, there still exists an onus on students to reveal more information than is required to secure their guaranteed accommodations. Disclosure over email and in one-on-one conversations with teaching staff and administrators can lead to cases where students feel obligated to describe their disabilities or psychiatric differences as a way to ensure access to their learning. The consequences of this process for many disabled and mad students are experiences of violence (for explanation of language choice, please see Titchkosky, 2001 and Reaume, 2002).

By violence, I refer to the institutional violence that is a result of having to engage in a system that relies on the uneven exchange of private and personal medical information for access to the necessary equipment and support to be successful in higher education. This violence is a consequence of the obscure, risky, and often complex nature of the disclosure process for disabled and mad students who are transitioning from high school or who have acquired an impairment or diagnosis during their time in higher education. Understanding this process is often necessary for their success in this sometimes-violent space ... More importantly, however, students should be aware that there are opportunities to subvert these violent processes by working collaboratively with faculty to ensure access to their education. Faculty and administrators, too, should acknowledge their role in maintaining this violence and work towards dismantling it to be replaced with other possibilities.

Similar to the experiences of those I interviewed for my research, many of my experiences of disclosure in higher education were violent (Shanouda, 2019). They include differential treatment where professors, instead of teaching assistants, grade my work; disability officers denying my requests for accommodations "because," they would say, "I had already made it this far without them"; and, administrators requiring new psycho-educational assessments, although my disability is permanent and my paperwork was up-to-date. In addition to these more serious experiences, I also navigated accusations made by teaching staff and disability service officers that I was malingering or lying, and they made attempts to limit the number of accommodations I could ask for. In the process of collecting data for my research project, I discovered that these experiences are almost pervasive.

What follows is a collection of narratives and quotes from disabled and mad students on their experiences of disclosure, passing, and coming out (Shanouda, 2019). For purposes of anonymity, I have used the following pseudonyms: Irene, Moana, Jimmy, Evadnae, Fernando, Theresa, Charlie and Quinn. Their narratives, presented as tightly constructed stories, provide readers with layers of information, such as the connections between experiences, as well as the consequences those experiences had on them as students. These stories challenge current practices around disclosure and demand a critical reflection of those practices. They illustrate how the requirement for disclosure opens up a space for violent interactions in higher education. These stories also describe both the immediate and on-going consequences of disclosure to both visibly and non-visibly disabled and mad students. In addition to the emotional and physical toll of experiencing violence, the consequences of disclosure for many participants were severe—with some dropping courses, others changing programs, and one student (from those quoted below) dropping out for a year. These students, however, also describe how they questioned the current process and pushed back to ensure their continued presence in higher education.

Disabled and mad students entering academia, or those who will acquire an impairment or diagnosis during their time in higher education, need to understand the potentially harmful impact that disclosure may have on them. Not all interactions will be violent, but some will and these interactions will stay with them, as they have for the participants I interviewed. The interactions will inform their understanding of disability and madness and shape how, when, where, and to whom they will feel comfortable sharing their story of difference. As a student, there is creative potential to undermine this process, subvert the requirements, and challenge the accommodations structure in higher education. Doing so means finding allies and champions amongst members of the teaching staff and in the administration. However, it is also the responsibility of faculty and staff to make themselves known to students by "calling-out" the violence of disclosure in their departments, faculties, in the classroom and by working alongside students to remove the requirement for disclosure in higher education.

REQUIRING DISCLOSURE: A VIOLENT PROCESS

Irene's narrative encapsulates how disclosure is an inherently violent process in higher education. Whilst finalizing a modification for their qualifying exam (or comprehensive exam), Irene was forced to disclose intimate experiences from her childhood:

> The accommodations requested seemed reasonable to everyone involved—their supervisor, committee members, their peers, the department administration—everyone. Except, in order to sanction the modification, Irene would have to go through Accessibility Services. Irene says the department needed some backup, "[…] need[ed] the paperwork." Bureaucratic desire led to real consequences. Irene's therapist was not accepted as a reference by the disability service officer—something to do with their professional title. It did not seem to matter that this was Irene's choice of referee and that this therapist could speak expertly to their need for specific modifications. Therefore, Irene was forced; to see a general practitioner (GP), who would then refer her to a psychologist or a therapist who could sign off on the paperwork. During her appointment, Irene was forced to disclose intimate experiences of childhood sexual violence. In exchange, Irene received three extra days to complete the exam.

Irene relayed this incident and argued that this "process [of disclosure] was kind of re-traumatizing." In addition to illustrating how the disclosure process can lead to experiences of violence and trauma, Irene's narrative also demonstrates that accommodations are often simple requests—extensions, extra time, assignment modifications; requests that can often be managed in the classroom or among a group of trained faculty members. Accommodation requests can become unnecessarily complicated however—as in Irene's case—when the demand for medical and bureaucratic approval is disproportionate to the request (Samuels, 2014). Irene had to tell her story in exchange for 3-extra days—a modification that could be granted without having to engage with the university's mandated policies. The exchange of information for access, in this example, as in many, is unfairly skewed.

The consequences of the disclosure process, however, are not always immediate. Moana's narrative illustrates how she experienced various violent consequences throughout the semester after disclosing to a professor before the start of class.

> I met her [a female academic] in December—a month before the class was meant to start. I thought I was being proactive and responsible. She didn't seem to see it that way. I told her about my disability—anxiety, heart condition, learning disability, etc. She seemed annoyed—or something like that. She kept asking me, "What do you want me to do about it?" She followed that up with, "You can't be missing class because this is an acting course." I thought, "Who said anything about missing class?" It seemed to me that she didn't really understand her role in this process. The class was hell. I was constantly frustrated—often tearing up—unsure of her requests or direction. She threatened me in front of the whole class. She would yell, "I can take your acting card away." I was scared after this point. I continued going to class, but things were weird, tense, and generally unpleasant moving forward. I was upset because I felt like I was letting her down. Her parting gift to me, and only me, was a personal assessment. To sum it up, she suggested that I quit acting. Her exact words were, "You should reconsider your future in this field."

In disclosing, Moana did not secure her accommodations nor was the classroom made more accessible. Instead, immediately after she disclosed, Moana was characterized as indolent—"you can't be missing class"—and throughout the semester she was threatened, yelled at, and told to change careers. Disclosure, as illustrated by Moana's quote, is not just a single encounter a student has with their professor or teaching assistant, but can be an on-going process that has a long-lasting effect.

Both Irene's and Moana's disabilities are non-visible. Students with non-visible disabilities have a more challenging time disclosing disability because their unrecognizable differences require them to meet a higher burden of proof (Samuels, 2003). However, the violence of disclosure—its violent consequences—also impact visibly disabled students. After having neck surgery to remove a mass, Jimmy's teaching assistant denied him an extension. Jimmy then visited the teaching assistant:

> Jimmy: It was such a nightmare. He was so ... I don't want to say hostile, but he just like ... it just seemed like every time I opened my mouth or sent him an email I was like personally going out of my way to inconvenience him, when in fact I was doing everything I could do to be like the most ... meek and mild-mannered. And I'm already a fairly mild-mannered person, but like I was trying to be ... I was trying to be as small as I possibly could. Like this little mouse that they would have pity on and give an extension. But it eventually got to a point where I actually had to go this TA's office while I still had a drainage tube in my neck. [...] This tube, with like fluid draining out of my neck. It was definitely, it was like physically uncomfortable ... But like I had to go down to [school] and talk to him. And he was like, "Write a little blurb to me about why you're requesting an additional extension." And I was like, "Fine. I'll do that." And I went to great detail just to kind of like make a point, like do you really need to know ...

Disclosure is therefore also a part of visibly disabled and mad students experiences in higher education. They too have to be "authenticated" by the institution by handing in paperwork and registering, even though their differences are visibly apparent. Jimmy, under these circumstances, compounded with the stress of keeping up with classes and the extensions granted on other work, dropped out of school for the year. Having to leave school was a significant consequence. A consequence that is potentially overlooked by institutions because, unlike Jimmy, some students never return (O'Keeffe, 2013).

A SYSTEMIC VIOLENCE

Experiences of violence during disclosure are not limited to the classroom setting. Evadnae describes below, disability service officers and the intake process itself can be a distressing experience (Goode, 2007). Evadnae explains here what it means to have disability service officers advise her to drop her courses after she sought support:

> "When I got my first intake when the ... person I spoke to was just like, "Yeah. So, have you considered dropping some of your courses?" And I'm like, "No. Why would I consider that?" And then she was just like, "Well, like I think that might be better for you." I'm like, "I didn't come in here for your opinion on what ... might be better for me. Like, I know what I'm doing. I just feel like this office should try to aid me in that, in trying to accomplish my goals. And I understand that there is a particular negotiation with taking on more than you can handle." [...] Or the emails that stand out the most for me from [disability service offices] is like, "Make sure you drop those courses. Make sure you like, you know, do it before the deadline so like xyz doesn't happen." And I'm just like, I don't think that this is the right approach, but I mean ...."

Counsellors or advisors are meant to help, provide support and guide students through higher education. However, Evadnae's experience demonstrates the focus is not on creating a more accessible and inclusive environment for diverse learners but rather on molding the individual to fit into a preconceived notion of what constitutes a successful student (Shanouda, 2019). The construction of this "normal" student influences disabled and mad student's self-perception and is possibly the most severe personal consequence that results from having to engage in the disclosing process. Here Fernando explains how these normative ideals influence him:

> "Being told you're inadequate by a system that seems like it's not built for you to the point where you start to think, "Well this is so entrenched that it can't possibly be wrong." So, therefore, there must be something wrong with me ... and sure there was something wrong, perhaps. [...] Like who wants to admit that they need extra help in a class. You're supposed to ... You're a university student. You're supposed to like have your shit together.

> You're supposed to be smart. You're supposed to be conscientious. You should be lucky that you're in that—you should feel lucky that you're in that classroom. But I wouldn't say that I was the problem. I would say that it was a problem of the systemic barrier that was the big issue. [...] We need to myth bust the representation of the normal student."

Fernando describes how disabled and mad students might feel as a result of having to navigate and disclose in a system that defines their way of being and learning as inadequate. Having to disclose in an environment, such as this, means that very few encounters lead to anything other than experiences of violence. Fernando also starts another important conversation in this statement: that moving forward means acknowledging that this normative context exists and that students and administrators need to work together to address the harmful consequences of the current system.

SUBVERTING DISCLOSURE

Disabled and mad students have always found ways of subverting the disclosure process and accompanying requests for "the paperwork." Participants indicated that they learned early on in their academic careers that when they revealed more information than what is considered appropriate they could avoid these requests. Theresa explains how this process was still violent, but that at the very least it meant she could avoid the bureaucratic hassle:

> "And then yeah, a lot of times I found the only way to get extensions, or to get like a late withdrawal, or something, from a course was to disclose more than I was actually comfortable with. But it was the only way to really ... to really get it done. A lot of times in like ... yeah, if you say, "I had a suicide attempt," it's super shocking and its way more information than you necessarily want to put out there, but at least you won't have to be fighting about it for the next six months."

Some students have always subverted the disclosure process (Sierra-Zarella, 2005). Irene, whose story of gaining a 3-day extension for her comprehensive exam described above, had throughout her undergraduate and master's degrees arranged accommodations but almost always informally:

> "... [W]hen I've had exams I've been able to in previous degrees at other universities say "I have a real issue with the exams." And I've been able to have professors accommodate me through letting me do oral exams instead [...] Cause the process of sitting in a room and writing became more and more stressful. Yeah, and so I've been treated for eating disorders before, but not specifically for anxiety around exams. Just like general anxiety. But I hadn't ever needed to have this taken to the university. People had usually accommodated around circumstances and taken me for my word. [...] I don't know why there actually—why they require so much documentation? Like is this bureaucratic machine

that produces paper trails, right. But like I don't—it's not even clear to me at an administrative level why they need these things."

Teaching staff had found a way, outside the system to facilitate Irene's learning. Irene points to the current system as perplexing and questions its standards and regulations. Her story highlights how important it is that disabled and mad students coming into higher education have a detailed understanding of the system. With this knowledge, students can start to question the system. Charlie explains how this might work:

> I think the solution would be for me to question why things are the way they are. Like why does my program only [last] two years? Why are the courses structured in the way they are? Why isn't there just no deadline? Why isn't there courses you can take in July/August so then it doesn't matter when you take them? Like more flexibility so that it doesn't become ... who is getting what and "be all you need" to push for certain sort of things. Cause I wish there was a world where I wouldn't see myself as having to ask for accommodations and extra help for things, and more time. And having to explain things and then having to worry about things as well. Just having to worry ... Like having to like wonder if I'm going to get extensions? Having to like make sure that like my accommodations are up and renew them every year. I think of all this extra work ...

Charlie suggests disabled and mad students should push back against the normative structures in higher education that regulate who, where, when, and how we can disclose and request inclusion of our different ways of learning. Dismantling this structure by demanding explanations for it and working in different ways to subvert the system (such as getting accommodations without the paperwork) is essential. As members of a community, this process must be done alongside allies and champions of progressive, equitable change to higher education.

Disabled and mad students want faculty and administrators to play a significant role in moving the conversation about access forward. Charlie describes here what it would mean to have faculty members as allies in creating new ways of approaching disability and madness in higher education.

> But just like changing the way things operate and ... I feel like having profs as allies too. To show—like them being more vocal as well to advocate on your behalf. That way I don't feel like I have to fight the battle myself, or with other students too. Like for my one ... my one friend where she had issues with her practicum. She really rocked the boat in terms of like, she went to like these committees with her faculty and sort of explained her experiences. But like why does she have to have that burden on her? Like that can—that's a lot for her to have. Why isn't it more of a collective process where we're all talking about it and we're all sort of pushing for change? Why does she have to hold all the risk?

When participants did find allies among the teaching staff—those that upload their slides, allow students to record lectures, to use accessible technology in the classroom (i.e., no laptop bans), those that describe images, use large font, contrasting colors, caption videos, and those who understand the unnecessary hurdles of the disclosure process—they stick with them. Quinn describes what some of these professors are doing and why it is important:

> Like I had a professor for a few courses that like … he knew what was sort of happening [student was in crisis]. And he was like, you know "We can modify assignments for you. Like we can, you know, like waive an assignment if you can't do it." Like he was, you know "You just have to let me know and we can work around this." So that was like really great to have that. … [H]e generally cares about his students. And it's not like … like it's not about having the documentation. […] You know, like if you're struggling I don't want to add to that. […] But I feel like, I don't know, like he gives his students as much … —like as many chances to succeed as possible. Which I think is what a teacher should be doing.

Quinn opened up to this professor, and the response was not violent, but caring—and included options for changing the assignments and rearranging parts of the course to ensure Quinn's successful involvement. While such arrangements may not be possible in every discipline or field of study, surely conversations about how to make classrooms and learning more accessible can take place in every corner of the institution. If disclosure more often led to this type of exchange, students would have very little concern about describing their differences to faculty. Administrators would do well to remember this exchange when creating new disclosure policies and regulations. It is important to consider what can be done to ensure a similar response every time a student discloses.

CONCLUSION

Critical and pedagogically minded instructors are those who are working to dismantle the disclosure process by restructuring curriculum design to reflect more accurately those who are in their classrooms. The violence of disclosure is not only a contemporary problem in higher education, but rather is a consequence of centuries of exclusion of women, Black, Indigenous, queer and trans people and, of course, disabled and mad people (Dolmage, 2017; Shanouda, 2019). Undoing this violence means reconciling this history. It means moving towards a more universal design of learning—one that is accessible and equity driven.

Those experiencing violence as a consequence of disclosure need to tell someone, have the violence recorded and call the experience violence. This advice, in many ways, is antithetical to what has been argued throughout this chapter—that disclosing personal information in higher education is harmful. I am not advising you to disclose disability when telling your story, but to ensure that there are witnesses to your experiences of violence. I have heard, too often, from disabled students, including those in my study, that these violent exchanges were "part of the deal" of being a disabled or mad student in a highly competitive academic setting. Students must move away from this line of thinking because violence, of any kind, should never be part of the learning process. Tell your story to someone you trust.

If your disability service officer is supportive, tell them, and ask for your story to be recorded in your file. If you have a good relationship with an instructor, ask them for support, especially if the violence is taking place in their department. Consider visiting the many other places in most universities where students can visit to have these harmful exchanges recorded—equity or human rights offices, offices of the ombudsperson and even certain student unions or disability-centric student groups can do this work. Finally, and most importantly, share these stories with other disabled and mad students at your institution and beyond—much like we are doing in writing this book together. In sharing our experiences, we can expect two outcomes: Firstly, we realize these violent experiences are all too common and that the problem is not our different ways of learning, but that of an ableist and sanist education system and secondly, that institutions of higher education can no longer ignore the problem that disclosure causes or write it off as anecdotal.

The participants narratives highlighted above, illustrate subversion of the disclosure process altogether which other students can learn from. Work with faculty who seem supportive to negotiate ways to include your learning and that allows you to avoid the bureaucracy. This is not your responsibility and there is always the looming threat that if granted it may be revoked at any point, and so do this work knowing there are limits and consequences.

Disabled and mad students are not asking for more than what is already guaranteed to them by law and what so much of the scholarship of teaching and learning has indicated is best practice (Dolmage, 2017; Price, 2014). Dismantling the disclosure process is a key step in implementing accessible education because if institutions of higher education do not require disclosure, then the system will have to be accessible from the start. Accessible education, oriented by equity and designed universally, allows students to focus on their learning and to avoid the violence that disclosure potentially brings.

REFERENCES

Cheuk, F. (2012). Locked closets and fishbowls: Self-disclosing disabilities. *Critical Disability Discourses/Discours Critiques Dans Le Champ du Handicap*, 4.

Dolmage, J. (2017). *Academic ableism: Disability and higher education*. Ann Arbor, MI: University of Michigan Press.

Goode, J. (2007). "Managing" disability: Early experiences of university students with disabilities. *Disability & Society, 22*(1), 35–48.

Kerschbaum, S. L., Eisenman, L. T., & Jones, J. M. (2017). *Negotiating disability disclosure and higher education*. Ann Arbor, MI: University of Michigan Press.

Matthew, N. (2009). Teaching the "invisible" disabled students in the classroom: Disclosure, inclusion and the social model of disability. *Teaching in Higher Education, 14*(3), 229–239.

O'Keeffe, P. (2013). A sense of belonging: Improving student retention. *College Student Journal, 47*(4), 605–613.

Olney, M. F., & Brockelman, K. F. (2003). Out of the disability closet: Strategic use of perception management by select university students with disabilities. *Disability & Society, 18*(1), 35–50.

Price, M. (2014). *Mad at school: Rhetorics of mental disability and academic life*. Ann Arbor, MI: University of Michigan Press.

Reaume, G. (2002). Lunatic to patient to person: Nomenclature in psychiatric history and the influence of patients' activism in North America. *International Journal of Law and Psychiatry, 25*(4), 405–426.

Samuels, E. (2003). My body, my closet: Invisible disability and the limits of coming out discourse. *GLQ: A Journal of Lesbian and Gay Studies, 9*, 223–255.

Samuels, E. (2014). *Fantasies of identification: Disability, gender, race*. New York, NY: New York University Press.

Shanouda, F. (2019). *The politics of passing: Disabled and mad students' experiences of disclosure in higher education* (Doctoral Dissertation).

Sierra-Zarella, E. (2005). Adapting and "passing": My experiences as a graduate student with multiple invisible disabilities. In L. Ben-Moshe, R. C. Cory, M. Feldbaum, & K. Sagendorf (Eds.), *Building pedagogical curb cuts: Incorporating disability in the university classroom and curriculum* (pp. 139–146). Syracuse, NY: The Graduate School, Syracuse University.

Titchkosky, T. (2001). Disability: A rose by any other name?: "People-first" language in Canadian society. *Canadian Review of Sociology/Revue Canadienne de Sociologie, 38*, 125–140.

CHAPTER 6

Negotiating the Space of Academia as a Disabled Student

LEECHIN HENG

INTRODUCTION

My job in life is not to educate you about disability. But Ok, there was one instance where it was that bad that I had to do something. We had this "showtime" called "research hub." PhD students are shoulder tapped to present about their studies, mostly of their research about disabled people. One time, someone presented their study about disabled students. As usual, the focus was on themselves and the able-bodied fight to advocate for disabled students to go to school, and so on. Out of the blue, during their presentation, they showed a photo of a disabled student in a wheelchair with an able-bodied person "helping" to push them to school or something like that. This exemplified an epic representation of the martyr and Tiny Tim. I kept my silence as usual at yet another presentation that reproduces disabled people as vulnerable. But the next day, a disabled friend of mine "grumbled" about their own personal Tiny Tim experiences on the social media site which I shared with the research hub group. And the presenter, strangely enough, texted me to say she got the message. But their attitude towards me after that was one where I should have remained silent like I always had done.

This chapter reflects on the seemingly common occurrence of disabled students finding themselves alone surrounded by able-bodied colleagues and academics in the area of their study, department, or even the whole college. It can be both an isolating and infuriating experience—especially when it comes to matters relating to disability or experiences of marginalisation—to be the elephant in the room as the only person who has experienced the topic of discussion, rather than hypotheses and assumptions based on the experiences of others. Yet, there is an implicit pressure to maintain what must remain unchallenged in the academy (Slee, 2011). This often had me biting my tongue over the assumed incompetence that had often been constructed on disabled people at the same time that able-bodied colleagues and academics construct themselves to be the voice and the champion of the vulnerable.

This chapter explores the fine lines, or what runs between the lines, of the knowledge that is accepted as given in the academy. My research interests led me to explore the development and facilitation of a new initial teacher education (ITE) programme that aspires to make education inclusive and equitable to historically marginalised students. Purcell (2012) states that "whoever controls space … also controls what can and cannot happen" in this space. My doctoral study explores what can and cannot be said in relation to how inclusion is understood and practiced in teacher education. Likewise, this chapter explores the finer lines of what can and cannot be questioned in the academy.

The chapter starts with an investigation of the transition between being physically excluded from mainstream schooling as a disabled child, to being included into the space of higher education later in life. It then discusses the liminality, or disorientation, of becoming a researcher and negotiating among people that claim to be the voice of those marginalised, while critically reflecting on how these voices continued to be stifled. Lastly, it discussed the negotiation of learning the implicit rules of being a disabled student in the academic space. The chapter suggests ways that the academy can break away from the system that is governing how the academic space is organised, so that it can realise its rhetoric of nurturing the leaders of tomorrow, including those with disabilities.

PERSONAL AND POLITICAL IDENTITY

My doctoral study explores the development of a new initial teacher education (ITE) programme to address ongoing disparities in educational outcomes. The core focus of this study was to inquire into how teacher educators in this programme attempt to challenge existing educational approaches that have worked well for some students, at the expense of those who do not identify with the dominant—white, middle-class, heterosexual, able-bodied—culture (Bishop et al., 2009; Macfarlane et al., 2008; Slee, 2011). The study speaks to me in two ways. Firstly, as someone who was excluded from the gate of special and mainstream schooling as a child in Malaysia, the opportunity to explore the making-of an ITE programme that aspires to make education inclusive to all children, seemed a godsend. Yet, now that I am included into the gate of higher education, I understand Graham and Slee's (2006) adage that "to include is not necessarily to *be* inclusive" (p. 3, emphasis in original). What I found myself *overcoming* and perhaps still *struggling to overcome*, in academic culture was conforming to what is not written in the acceptance letter into this implicit (able-bodied) culture of a higher education institution.

As a person who was home schooled, conformations to institutional structures or schooling practices—such as putting on uniforms that represent my gender, school or educational level—were all unfamiliar to me. Although many aspects of this rigid structure are not explicit in higher education culture, this does not mean that universities are not ordered by implicit sets of rules that govern how things should be organised and how social actors within this institutional culture should represent itself (Doerr, 2009). In lieu of the uniforms that regulate how I should perform my gender and cognitive ability, what awaits in the academy are tags that say *disabled student, international student, non-English native speaker*, and the list goes on. What was represented in all of these tags was the constructions of *difference* (from an implicit norm) that continue to "silo" students to conform to distinctive categories of difference.

This can create a feeling of isolation. Having more than one tag does not mean disabled students are spoilt for choice in getting to choose which *tag* among the many they want to belong. Disabled students may either constantly find themselves negotiating or confined to identify with certain tags, or they are made to feel that they would feel more comfortable with other tags. Belonging has also been a topic of much discussion in disability studies. Research has pointed out how the reason which teachers and schools often give for rejecting students identified as *different* is that these students belong somewhere else (Baglieri, 2017; Black-Hawkins & Florian, 2012). This suggests that there should be a space that can adequately accommodate the *special needs* of disabled students. Even though neither teachers nor schools know where and if such a space exists, what is explicit is that these students do not belong to the particular teachers' classroom or schooling practices.

On the same note, disabled students often find themselves being directed by staff in academic and student support departments at universities to an assumed space where they can receive the adequate support they need. For example, making the study place more functional for disabled students can be assumed as the most important concern of the academy in order to enable students to succeed in their academic journey. Many disabled students find that what really tires them in their research journey is not their study but getting through the bureaucracies of the most basic accommodations that will make their study environment more functional for them. It can be assumed that the more tags disabled students receive in the academy means the more *additional* support they are entitled to receive from the university. However, what is often the case is that disabled students can find themselves being endlessly directed to various departments in the hope that one of them will have the solution on how best to accommodate the disabled students' *special needs* in the academy. In the end, the support they actually receive is not more than what their able-bodied colleagues receive as a given, such as a study space with a desk and computer.

THE POLITICS OF VOICE IN RESEARCH

What guided my research was a strong desire to stay away from yet another study that proclaimed to be the voice of the vulnerable or aimed to improve on the lives of *people like me*. As someone living with a rare genetic condition, and a very visible disability, I have participated in numerous medical and scientific research projects with that aim. These were, as Oliver called it, most definitely a "rape model of research" (Oliver, 1992, p. 109) for the way able-bodied researchers *extorted* insights from the experiences and life stories shared by disabled participants to advance their own status in the academy, while the lot of disabled people's lives still remained the same as before the research began.

Although the emergence of disability studies has generated much critiques on this so-called "rape model" (Garland-Thomson, 2002; Linton, 1998, 2005; Mertens et al., 2011; Oliver, 2013), it cannot be assumed that researchers who claim to have lived experiences of disability, either through the experiences of having a relative or a child with a disability, are not *at risk* of stifling the voices of disabled people. A question which disability studies scholars such as O'Toole (2013) frequently ask about these truth or experience claims, is: *What is your relationship with disability?* As much of the literature on disability studies has pointed out, effects of marginalisation is different for those born with impairments and those who acquire them later in life (Linton, 2007; O'Toole, 2013). For a nondisabled family member, these effects differ in relation to their proximity with the disabled family member. When people attempt to speak for others, they need to be aware of the usefulness of what they say. After all, their presumptions of what living with disabilities is like can be very different from what it is to those who experience its effects on a daily basis.

Nonetheless, the experience of finding yourself as the only person with a disability surrounded by able-bodied peers and academics is not unusual. As Megan Conway (2012), the managing editor of the Review of Disability Studies Journal writes, "As a deaf-blind person who received her doctorate in Special Education from an esteemed university … I thought it was weird that I was the only one with a disability in my doctoral cohort—no, make that my entire doctoral program" (p. 3). Similarly, being the only student researcher in the field of inclusive education at my university meant I was among able-bodied peers and academics who purport to give voice to marginalised groups. This involved constantly negotiating between the two worlds of *hearing* able-bodied colleagues in the academy proclaiming to be martyrs for the voiceless, and *hearing* laments from their fellow peers in the disability community of the martyrs in the academy who silenced their voices instead of raising them. Sitting between these two identities was a frustrating experience, to say the least. What was infuriating is listening to how people create an assumed *other* in order to illustrate their own able-bodiedness. Such representation of able-bodiedness—or in being able to speak with their mouths—often justifies them as responsible for being the voice of those who cannot speak.

The insights which disabled students carry with them can be both a blessing, and a curse. The upside is that disabled people have first-hand knowledge not only about experiences of marginalisation—which saves them a lot of effort in trying to create an *other* and construct their research identity as martyrs for these vulnerable groups. Most of them also have first-hand experience of knowing what it feels like to be made the subject of research yet being spoken *of* as an object that is static and fix, rather than a full-bodied human being. However, the downsides, are also all that. Disabled students often have to be harsh on themselves in making sure that they are not exploiting their *power* as researchers, like their able-bodied colleagues, to extort or silence the voices of their disabled peers. In other words, they are constantly being critical of their own research position of whether their aspiration to the voices of the *unheard* is to contribute to the inclusion and emancipation of those voices in society (Annamma et al., 2016). Or, are those voices further silenced, intentionally or unintentionally, as the researcher aspires to advance their own academic goals (Harvey, 2013).

Although their status may change from that of being research subjects to researchers, it does not mean disabled students have more *power* to control the experiences of marginalisation in which they are situated. On the contrary, in order to be recognised as a member of research communities, they often have to suppress their thoughts and conform to assumptions of their able-bodied peers and academics. Even if they do not join in the chorus of these truth or experience claims, by keeping quiet, they are crudely reminded of their role to speak up against these voices that reproduce the status quo, rather than to mitigate existing inequities in society.

BEING A MARGINALISED RESEARCHER

The opportunity to explore a teacher education programme that aspired to include not just most or some but *all* children in the education system was inviting. Inclusion was certainly a *material*—or a research interest—that speaks to me. It is also a matter that a disabled researcher negotiates every minute and every second of their lives. Researching a subject that speaks directly to the marginalised researcher, as a topic like inclusion does, should be exciting and highly rewarding (Romano, 2004). Nevertheless, it can also be astoundingly exhausting. It is a situation which academic supervisors may find perplexing. It may be the first time they have supervised a topic that is personally related to their students' experiences, not just a topic of which both able-bodied supervisors and students can only claim to *speak* on behalf of. The different perspectives, or the real rather than assumed experiences of marginalisation, can potentially cause conflict between disabled students and their academic supervisors who may have never had their assumptions or truth claims challenged before.

Disciplinary knowledge in academia has often been critiqued as *fixed*, and therefore *accepted* as given (McPhail & Rata, 2016). Moreover, educationalists have often touted traditional ways of teaching to be suggestive of banking these so-called fixed knowledge into all students (Freire, 2005; Gilbert, 2013). In my research, I was critically aware of my position as a student researcher who was independent, amiable, and noticeably impaired enough to allow people to *feel good* about their openness to accepting difference. As a third generation, Chinese Malaysian, female, non-native English speaker, international student, middle class, wheelchair-user, and many yet-to-be identified identities, I was also aware that my diverse characteristics would traditionally qualify me in the role of research subject, rather than that of researcher.

I considered myself a *marginalised insider* in my research as I constantly had to remind myself to keep to my role of a researcher with an "approachable difference, just atypical enough to inspire without being off-putting" (Scott, 2013, p. 103). Being able to share my subjective knowledge of inclusion and experiences of marginalisation as a disabled student aided me to *enter* into somewhat reciprocal relationships with my participants. For example, at my interviews with them, my participants would talk about their experiences of marginalisation which they wondered if their colleagues have experiences of, even though these colleagues theorise about in their teaching. Such statements suggest their ease at talking about their own experiences to someone they feel safe and assured would understand experiences of marginalisation, even if our experiences may be different. My position as a disabled researcher legitimatised my presence in this research as a doctoral student interested in the aspiration of inclusion, but that was not enough on its own. Whether disabled students undertake research in the social sciences or the hard sciences, it is necessary for them to position themselves as independent yet *disabled* enough to allow able-bodied peers and academics to feel good about the openness of their department, or even academy, in accepting someone who is *different* from them. In my research I felt I had to ease my participants' and academic supervisors' acceptance of my presence in the academy, as the only acceptable way to encourage them to deflect from their presumptions of what living with disability is like.

Intended or otherwise, disabled students who plan to embark on research journeys of their own need to understand that their presence as researchers in institutional spaces dominated by able-bodied academics can at times cause uneasiness (Conway, 2012; Garland-Thomson, 2002; Scott, 2013). This discomfort is often constructed as a result of the *inappropriate* and *objectionable* behaviour of disabled students, and the onus is put on disabled students to ensure that they do not disrupt the culture, or the unquestioned truth claims about knowledge entrenched in the academy. While universities may purport to generate future researchers with the confidence to give voice and transform social ills and make the world a better place, students are nevertheless obliged to conform to the implicit regimes that continue to regulate how social actors are to conduct themselves. In my own four-year research journey, the steepest learning curves were the ones of constant negotiations of learning to be a docile student who is just disabled and intelligent enough to contribute to the academy of her own experiences of disability, yet also knowing not to challenge the assumed *difference* that is constructed to make the able-bodied colleagues and academics to feel good about their ability to speak on behalf of the voiceless. Coming back to the narrative at the beginning of this chapter, it is hoped that the academy can one day become a space where students and academics can be open-minded and accepting of different and multiple worldviews—especially of the views and voices that have historically been marginalised in academy and society.

CONCLUSION

As scholars and researchers it is our obligation to ourselves and to the people who we profess to speak for to "always look for how we can improve things … [and to continually ask] how can we do it better" (Graham & Slee, 2006, p. 2). This chapter urges academic cultures to stop *labelling* students into fixed and accepted categories of difference and instead to engage with them as human beings with identities that are multiple and fluid. It demands able-bodied academics to step out of their comfort zones and to be prepared to accept *differences* and *dissonances* from disabled people who will no longer make their presence and voices heard in the academy *just* enough to make the academics *feel good* about themselves.

Why does the able-bodied academic *study* disability, and the experiences of those they can never really share? Just as the white heterosexual middle class male may have little ethical ground in studying or teaching about the experience of African American lesbians in ghettos, where is the ethical dialogue about the able-bodied academic making a career out of stifling the voices of those already rendered invisible in society, in order to exert their own? Earlier in the chapter, I mentioned that the academy does not need another research about disabled people's experiences written from the presumptive standpoint of yet another able-bodied researcher. Yet as Shildrick (2009) stresses, what academy needs are not works that further create a distinction between able-bodied vs. disabled bodies but a different way of thinking that "strive to exceed the very experience of boundaries" (p. 170). The academy has a lot to do to break away from the implicit schooling structure that governs academics and students in their respective roles as givers and receivers of knowledge to a create a space for questions and the co-constructions of ideas yet unthought.

REFERENCES

Annamma, S., Connor, D., & Ferri, B. (2016). Dis/ability critical race studies (discrit): Theorizing at the intersections of race and dis/ability. In D. Connor, B. Berri, & S. Annamma (Eds.), *DisCrit: Disability studies and critical race theory in education* (pp. 9–32). New York, NY: Teachers College Press.

Baglieri, S. (2017). *Disability studies and the inclusive classroom: Critical practices for embracing diversity in education* (2nd ed.). New York, NY: Routledge.

Bishop, R., Berryman, M., Cavanagh, T., & Teddy, L. (2009). Te Kotahitanga: Addressing educational disparities facing Māori students in New Zealand. *Teaching and Teacher Education*, *25*(5), 734–742. https://doi.org/10.1016/j.tate.2009.01.009

Black-Hawkins, K., & Florian, L. (2012). Classroom teachers' craft knowledge of their inclusive practice. *Teachers and Teaching*, *18*(5), 567–584. https://doi.org/10.1080/13540602.2012.709732

Conway, M. A. (2012, October 1). Editorial: A note from the mouse who wanted to be the farmer's wife, Editorial. *Review of Disability Studies: An International Journal*, *8*(3), 3–4. Retrieved from http://ezproxy.canterbury.ac.nz/login?url=http://search.ebscohost.com/login.aspx?direct=true&db=sih&AN=83408195&site=ehost-live

Doerr, N. M. (2009). *Meaningful inconsistencies: Bicultural nationhood, the free market, and schooling in Aotearoa New Zealand*. New York, NY: Berghahn Books.

Freire, P. (2005). *Education for critical consciousness*. New York, NY: The Continuum Publishing.

Garland-Thomson, R. (2002). Integrating disability, transforming feminist theory. *NWSA Journal*, *14*(3), 1–32.

Gilbert, J. (2013). What should initial teacher education programmes for 2022 look like and why? *Waikato Journal of Education*, *18*(1), 105–116.

Graham, L., & Slee, R. (2006). *Inclusion?* Paper presented at the American Educational Research Association (AERA) 2006 Annual Conference, San Francisco.

Harvey, J. (2013). Footprints in the field: Researcher identity in social research. *Methodological Innovations Online*, *8*(1), 86–98. Retrieved from http://mio.sagepub.com/content/8/1/86.abstract. https://doi.org/10.4256/mio.2013.0006

Linton, S. (1998). Disability studies/not disability studies. *Disability & Society*, *13*(4), 525–539.

Linton, S. (2005). What Is disability studies? *PMLA, 120*(2), 518–522. https://doi.org/10.2307/25486177

Linton, S. (2007). *My body politic: A memoir.* Ann Arbor, MI: The University of Michigan Press.

Macfarlane, A., Glynn, T., Grace, W., Penetito, W., & Bateman, S. (2008). Indigenous epistemology in a national curriculum framework? *Ethnicities, 8*(1), 102–126. https://doi.org/10.1177/1468796807087021

McPhail, G., & Rata, E. (2016). Comparing curriculum types: "Powerful knowledge" and "21st century learning." *New Zealand Journal of Educational Studies, 51*(1), 53–68. https://doi.org/10.1007/s40841-015-0025-9

Mertens, D., Sullivan, M., & Stace, H. (2011). Disability communities: Transformative research for social justice. In N. K. Denzin & Y. Lincoln (Eds.), *The Sage handbook of qualitative research 4th edition* (pp. 227–241). London, UK: Sage.

O'Toole, C. (2013). Disclosing our relationships to disabilities: An invitation for disability studies scholars. *Disability Studies Quarterly, 33*(2), 1–15.

Oliver, M. (1992). Changing the social relations of research production? *Disability, Handicap & Society, 7*(2), 101–114.

Oliver, M. (2013). The social model of disability: Thirty years on. *Disability & Society, 28*(7), 1024–1026. https://doi.org/10.1080/09687599.2013.818773

Purcell, R. (2012). Community development and everyday life. *Community Development Journal, 47*(2), 266–281.

Romano, T. (2004). *Crafting authentic voice.* Portsmouth, NH: Heinemann.

Scott, J. (2013). Problematizing a researcher's performance of "insider status": An autoethnography of "designer disabled" identity. *Qualitative Inquiry, 19*(2), 101–115. https://doi.org/10.1177/1077800412462990

Shildrick, M. (2009). *Dangerous discourses of disability, subjectivity and sexuality.* London, UK: Palgrave Macmillan.

Slee, R. (2011). *The irregular school: Exclusion, schooling and inclusive education.* New York, NY: Routledge.

CHAPTER 7

Disability Studies in Higher Education: Developing Identity and Community

MEGAN ZAHNEIS

INTRODUCTION

Why do students attend university? To learn a trade or pursue a passion, but also to learn who they are professionally and, perhaps more importantly, personally. They typically spend up to four or more years of early adulthood developing identity which includes discovering and affirming their personal beliefs and sense of self and learning to square their own self-perceptions with society's expectations (Baxter Magolda, 2014; Jones & Abes, 2013).

The notion of a college campus as the site of self-discovery as well as scholarly pursuits has become an important part of the pitch universities make to prospective students. In marketing and recruitment efforts, higher education professionals emphasize the student's journey of self-discovery equally with their school's academic prowess. They appeal to minority students in hopes of broadening their diversity portfolios and constructing affinity groups. Once these students arrive on campus, they are encouraged to explore their marginalized identities—whether through race, ethnicity, sexual orientation or gender—throughout their collegiate careers (Schuh et al., 2017). Yet disability is often not included among these forms of diversity, in higher education or in society at large. While disabled people comprise the world's largest minority population (Disability Statistics, 2018), disability is most often viewed as a marker of difference without any of the positive identity-forming traits of other minority populations. Disability is typically not treated as part of the identity-development process in higher education, but rather, as an obstacle needing accommodation (Kim & Aquino, 2017).

Students with disabilities should have the opportunity to explore disability as a facet of one's identity, to understand the academic and social contexts disability is situated within, and to gain exposure to the sense of community, culture and pride inherent in many who identify as disabled. Disability should be part of the identity-development journey that has cemented itself as one of the primary purposes of higher education.

That journey is one I have pursued for the past three years as a disabled undergraduate student, and one that has been propelled by my coursework in disability studies. I enrolled in an Introduction to Disability Studies course in my second year of school, and in doing so, found a vibrant form of academic inquiry—and a personal passion—that has shaped how I view myself and the world. This chapter explores the relationship of disability studies to the university experience. It stands as evidence that universities should provide students with academic programs in disability studies as a means of fostering disability identities and communities.

WHAT IS DISABILITY STUDIES?

Disability studies is an interdisciplinary academic perspective through which disability and the lived experience of disabled people are examined (Linton, 1998). The field emerged in the 1980s, and much of its scholarship is predicated on the social model of disability that emerged from the disability movement in the United Kingdom (UK). In contrast to the medical model of disability, which is most prominent in society at large, disability studies calls into question "the view of disability as an individual deficit or defect that can be remedied solely through medical intervention or rehabilitation by 'experts' and other service providers" (Society for Disability Studies, n.d.). Rejecting the notion that to be disabled is a pitiable and burdensome fate, the social model—and disability studies—instead treat disability as a social, political, cultural and economic phenomenon that affects all societies, pivoting "away from the functional limitations of impaired individuals onto the problems caused by disabling environments, barriers and cultures" (Barnes, 2003, p. 7).

Rather than a physiological problem inherent in an individual, the social model defines disability as the societal obstacles a person may face as a result of that bodily difference—whether the lack of an access ramp or an "ableist" remark. In the world of disability studies, disability is not inherently negative, but merely a marker of diversity. Disability studies and the social model construct disability as a minority identity, one that comes with positive and negative experiences. Disability, like any other minority, contains its own community, whose members often view it as a source of pride—dependent, as with any minority status, on their individual experiences with that identity.

Disability studies places a heavy emphasis on the voices of disabled people inside and out of the academy, considering them influencers of and contributors to the field's scholarship, as opposed to a subject of examination by non-disabled individuals. In a reversal of one troubling aspect of identity studies, disability studies allow the studied to become the studiers—and, indeed, the field demonstrates a dedication to centering the perspectives of disabled individuals. Its unique positioning within both academia and the "real world" means that disability studies can be applied in both theoretical and practical contexts; outside of the academy, disability studies work is also intertwined with the disability rights movement and disability culture.

It is useful to define disability studies by considering what it is not (Linton, 1998). Rather than focusing on accommodations and legal requirements, both of which are important, disability studies in the classroom transcends a deficiency-based approach by proposing a student-centered experience. Disability studies teaches that it is higher education, not the student, that must change (Linton, 1998).

MY JOURNEY WITH DISABILITY STUDIES

Disability has been a part of my identity from birth and I have always been relatively accepting of its role in my life. Yet prior to attending college and enrolling in an Introduction to Disability Studies course as a means of fulfilling a graduation requirement, I was unaware that disability was or could be a vehicle for intellectual and academic exploration, or a way for me to engage with my campus community on an intimate level. I discovered disability studies is both deeply personal and an academically grounded mode of introducing students to a community and identity they may not be aware existed. Although a still-developing field, with intersectional voices emerging (e.g., Schalk, 2017) and facing some critique of the categorization of identity (McRuer, 2006), disability studies can play a significant role in shaping the students' co-curricular and academic collegiate experience.

ACADEMIC WORK IN DISABILITY STUDIES

Enrolling in an Introduction to Disability Studies class marked the first time I felt I could contribute something to a classroom because of, and not in spite of, my disability. Within that classroom, I became a resident expert, a primary source of knowledge who could contribute personal experience to class discussions. Never before had I felt my disability was a truly additive facet of a classroom; instead, entrenched in a deficit-based model, I had felt my disability was a burden in need of accommodation by my instructors and peers. In disability studies, my perspective is valued and sought out. This changed the way I participate in the course.

I found myself engaging with disability studies course material in new ways. Reading the work of disability studies scholars, I felt understood, spurred by the knowledge that many had studied the experiences and feelings I thought I had been alone in having. Discovering the concept of "inspiration porn," wherein disabled people are often objectified as sources of motivation in mainstream media (Young, 2014) marked one such epiphany for me; notions like this one lent a scholarly credence to personal gripes I had always harbored but could never pinpoint why. Reading academic literature on disability often felt as if I were holding myself up to a mirror. Gaining a vocabulary and academic framework for describing my own life proved personally and academically fulfilling.

Disability studies has reframed the way I view my disability and, ultimately, myself and society. I grew up, as many disabled people do, enmeshed in the medical model of disability and surrounded by doctors and nurses who spoke to and of me in terms of diagnoses and symptoms. While these medical professionals were not doing so to denigrate me, and while I have been fortunate to receive excellent medical care throughout my life, I had not considered another schema existed through which I could see myself. … By introducing me to the social model, disability studies assisted to reposition my own mind. Just as it had within the dynamic of the classroom. I had never before been exposed to a scholarly perspective that presented disability as additive, a marker of diversity and not deficiency.

The notion of being worthy of accommodation, in society and at school, was one I knew I should accept, but was never thoroughly able to until encountering disability studies. Reading disability studies literature has prompted me to stop problematizing myself and instead to examine structural flaws in our society that present barriers for me. I have become more leery of the status quo of disability's place in society and, importantly, more willing to contribute to a paradigm shift in that role. Throughout my time in college, I have done so not only in terms of how I present myself as an individual—through my actions and writings—but also by becoming more involved in the disability advocacy community.

DISABILITY STUDIES AND CO-CURRICULAR INVOLVEMENT

Early in my collegiate career, I helped form a student group, grounded in disability studies concepts, which aims to be a voice for disabled students and to raise awareness of the lived experience of disability. As the number of students registered with my university's disability services office significantly grew, it sought to involve students more directly in the office's operations by establishing an advisory group. The group was originally conceived as a small group of student liaisons within the disability services office This group eventually became a university-recognized student organization called the Students with Disabilities Advisory Council (SDAC). Through faculty and student workshops, presentations at professional-development conferences and other awareness-centered initiatives, SDAC members act as self-advocates and as representatives of disability in the university community.

One of the priorities SDAC set at its inception was to introduce our campus to the theory underlying disability studies—namely, that disability is not inherently "a Bad Thing, capital B, capital T" (Young, 2014)—and to the idea that disability ought to be considered a facet of institutional and cultural diversity. Particularly, we were interested in engaging faculty members who in their professional lives typically only encounter disability in the context of students in need of accommodation (or, in other words, in terms of the medical model). Instead, we seek to humanize disability for faculty members, and offer our personal perspectives on what it is to be a college student with a disability.

The group was also designed as a peer-to-peer support structure, one that would allow students who are registered with the disability services office and/or identify as having a disability to connect with one another. My involvement in SDAC has served as a source of friendship and camaraderie with other members and with fellow disability studies students. These bonds, built on a mutual understanding, have been the strongest ones I have formed in college; in fact, they mark some of the most formative relationships I have ever forged. Put simply, these peers are able to empathize with and relate to me in ways that no one else in our campus community can. While these relationships have been a very significant part of my identity development, they are perhaps most objectively measured in the disability studies classroom, where I have for the first time been able to explore my identity with peers who, like me, are able to connect with the material on an intellectual and intimately personal level—peers with whom I have only to exchange a knowing look to know that they, too, "get it."

As co-president of SDAC, I have witnessed firsthand the sense of community disability studies fosters. One first-year student told me our group and the disability studies program at our university were among the primary reasons she chose to attend this school. This disabled first-year student entered college intending to develop her disability identity through coursework in disability studies and involvement with our student group, both of which have contributed to her sense of purpose and overall identity-development journey.

What if my situation and that of the first-year student were not an exception but the norm? What if more students were able to deliberately develop their own disability identities in higher education? What if, just as students of color may choose to attend a historically Black college or students who are part of the LBGTQ community might attend a liberal arts school with a tradition of supporting their identities, disabled students could similarly find a locus of support within their university?

Disability studies ought to be incorporated in universities' inclusive philosophies. Like the distinct disciplines which exist to examine other minority communities—such as African-American and queer studies—disability studies should be taught with careful attention to intersectionality and with the goal of fostering inclusive campus communities.

Although minority students of all identities face challenges in college, an established support system for disabled students—grounded in disability studies concepts—would play an instrumental role in their identity-development journeys. Indeed, the framework disability studies provides students and institutions for understanding disability is a perspective that should be afforded to everyone in higher education.

INCORPORATING DISABILITY STUDIES AT AN INSTITUTIONAL LEVEL

In an ideal world, every university would house a department or degree program for disability studies, and every college student could be exposed to the foundations of the field via a compulsory introductory course incorporated into the school's graduation requirements. It is time to make that world a reality. Universities can and should take strides toward a disability studies mindset.

In the absence of a full-fledged disability studies program, institutions can offer at least an introductory disability studies course to students. This course could count toward cultural competency and diversity requirements at liberal arts schools. Disability studies concepts can also be infused into general-education curriculum; as an interdisciplinary field, disability studies has real-life implications for every student, regardless of their chosen career path. For example, literature majors can study the works of disabled writers (Clare, 2017); premedical students would benefit from understanding the medical and social models of disability (Campbell, 2009, Wilson, 2000); law and political science students can examine the intersections of disability and public policy (Roulstone & Prideaux, 2012; Soldatic & Meekosha, 2014), preservice teachers can apply disability studies in their classrooms (Baglieri et al., 2011; Cosier & Ashby, 2016), business students can study the needs of a hugely diverse consumer contingency; those entering client-facing fields like social work and psychology gain important context for working with disabled people (Hiranandani, 2005; Shakespeare, 2005). Simply put, disability studies is not a "special-interest" field. It is relevant to every student.

Universities should include disability in their diversity statements and more broadly, in their definitions of diversity. Disability-specific programming and initiatives should be incorporated into the work of offices devoted to diversity affairs, and enrichment opportunities designated for diverse students should be made available to disabled students. Making explicit mention of disability in conversations about diversity not only acknowledges and honors the lived experience of an entire population, but also lets disabled students know that their perspectives are valued on an institutional level (Kim & Aquino, 2017).

Disability services offices at higher education institutions should adopt an inclusion mindset as opposed to a deficiency-based accommodation approach. In doing so, they might eliminate the stigma many students feel comes with registering as disabled. This would foster a greater sense of confidence and community in the students they serve, and perhaps even trigger in a few individuals the identity-development journey I have undergone.

If universities market themselves as pathways to and through identity development, then they owe it to their disabled students—and, indeed, to their able-bodied ones—to provide instruction in disability studies. For the disabled student, disability studies can be that deeply personalized and intellectually stimulating vehicle for self-discovery. Equally as affirming to a student is the knowledge that their university recognizes and celebrates their identity; disabled students deserve this institutional acknowledgement of disability as a minority identity. Through a disability studies curriculum, universities can provide students a space to explore that minority identity, to question societal perceptions of disability while defining and constructing their own relationship to it, and even to change the way disabled students perceive themselves and the world in which they live.

REFERENCES

Baglieri, S., Valle, J. W., Connor, D. J., & Gallagher, D. J. (2011). Disability studies in education: The need for a plurality of perspectives on disability. *Remedial and Special Education, 32*(4), 267–278.

Barnes, C. (2003, September 3). *Disability studies: What's the point?* Keynote address presented at Disability studies: Theory, policy and practice conference, University of Lancaster, UK.

Baxter Magolda, M. (2014). Self-Authorship. *New Directions for Higher Education, 2014*(166), 25–33.

Campbell, F. K. (2009). Medical education and disability studies. *Journal of Medical Humanities, 30*(4), 221–235.

Clare, E. (2017). *Brilliant imperfection: Grappling with cure.* Durham, NC: Duke University Press.

Cosier, M., & Ashby, C. (Eds.). (2016). *Enacting change from within: Disability studies meets teaching and teacher education.* New York, NY: Peter Lang.

Disability Statistics: Information, Charts, Graphs and Tables. (2018, June 22). Retrieved from https://www.disabled-world.com/disability/statistics/

Hiranandani, V. (2005). Towards a critical theory of disability in social work. *Social Work, 6*(1), 1–14.

Jones, S. R., & Abes, E. S. (2013). *Identity development of college students: Advancing frameworks for multiple dimensions of identity.* San Francisco, CA: Jossey-Bass.

Kim, E., & Aquino, K. C. (Eds.). (2017). *Disability as diversity in higher education: Policies and practices to enhance student success.* New York, NY: Routledge.

Linton, S. (1998). *Claiming disability: Knowledge and identity.* New York, NY: New York University Press.

McRuer, M. (2006). *Crip theory: Cultural signs of queerness and disability.* New York, NY: New York University Press.

Roulstone, A., & Prideaux, S. (2012). *Understanding disability policy.* Bristol, UK: Policy Press.

Schalk, S. (2017). Critical disability studies as methodology. *Lateral, 6*(1).

Schuh, J. H., Jones, S. R., & Torres, V. (Eds.). (2017). *Student services: A handbook for the profession.* San Francisco, CA: Jossey-Bass.

Shakespeare, T. (Ed.). (2005). *The disability reader: Social science perspectives.* London, UK: Continuum.

Soldatic, K., & Meekosha, H. (Eds.). (2014). *The global politics of impairment and disability: Processes and embodiments.* London, UK: Routledge.

Wilson, J. C. (2000). Making disability visible: How disability studies might transform the medical and science writing classroom. *Technical Communication Quarterly, 9*(2), 149–161.

Young, S. (2014, April). *I'm not your inspiration, thank you very much* [Video file]. Retrieved from https://www.ted.com/talks/stella_young_i_m_not_your_inspiration_thank_you_very_much

PART II

ADJUSTMENTS FOR LEARNING AND CONTRIBUTING

CHAPTER 8

Beyond Compliance: Disabled Student Activism on Campus

JUSTIN FREEDMAN, LAURA JAFFEE, KATIE ROQUEMORE, YOSUNG SONG AND HETSIE VEITCH

INTRODUCTION

Our group, the Beyond Compliance Coordinating Committee (BCCC), was founded in 2001 by graduate students with disabilities and allies at Syracuse University in the United States. Going beyond compliance means implementing structural changes to make campuses accessible—for disabled people, people of color, for poor, trans*,
[i] queer, undocumented, and Indigenous folks, and all those at the intersections—not just meeting minimum requirements to comply with legal obligations. It is a social justice approach to disability that is "based in the belief that people's abilities and rights to contribute to and benefit from higher education are not dependent on their bodies or psyches conforming to dominant norms" (Evans et al., 2017, p. x). In the words of disabled activist Alice Wong (2018), "accessibility is more than just adherence to a law. It's an ethos that values different ways of being in the world" (para. 9).

The BCCC uses critical theories of disability as a framework for campus activism aimed at changing campus culture and disability policies and to conceptualize a move beyond "simple compliance to the law mindset" (Cory et al., 2010, p. 30). Critical theories examine the material impact of economic, political and social policy on the lived experiences of disabled people and urge us to reassess the ableist normativity that is entrenched in our societies. They challenge the over-simplified binary thinking about disability and foreground the representation and participation of disabled people in all aspects of society (Meekosha & Shuttleworh, 2009; Shildrick, 2012). Our work is guided by the belief that meaningful participation for students with disabilities cannot be achieved by providing the minimum level of access nor without challenging the status quo (Broderick & Lalvani, 2017). We insist that disability should be ingrained in the institutional culture of the university and not a mere afterthought when "diversity groups" are considered. Consequently, the presence and participation of disabled students, staff and faculty in ALL aspects of campus life is imperative.

In the U.S., colleges and universities must meet specific legal compliance for mandates of non-discrimination and reasonable accommodations for students who identify as having disabilities. Section 504 of the Rehabilitation Act (1975), for example, requires that institutions that receive federal funding provide reasonable accommodations for students with disabilities; the Americans with Disabilities Act (ADA) (1990) mandates that public entities, such as colleges and universities, cannot deny students admission or participation because of their disability (Shallish, 2017). Private institutions that accept federal funding in the form of student financial aid and research grants are also mandated to not discriminate against students with disabilities (DaDeppo, 2009). Despite these laws, disabled students encounter myriad barriers to meaningful participation on campus, including access problems in classes and for campus events and student activities.

The BCCC works within and beyond the current laws to advocate for our university to create structures and develop attitudes that ensure meaningful participation in ways that the law cannot. This is true for students in the U.S., just as it is true for students with disabilities in other countries. When we advocate for "beyond compliance," we are advocating for more than superficial nods towards diversity and inclusion from colleges and universities. "Beyond compliance" values disabled lives with the recognition of disability as a form of diversity that enriches our university community (Kim & Aquino, 2017).

This chapter expands the discussion on compliance. It looks at action in approaches to disability student activism. The chapter discusses some of the limitations of advocacy work within institutions that prioritize profit and are premised on the replication of disability injustice. It offers, through practical examples, warnings as to how "compliance" can sometimes be used for more selfish gains. Based on the challenges we have faced the final section suggests how to more effectively work beyond compliance in higher education through collective action and activism.

RECENT STUDENT ADVOCACY

A major point of advocacy for the BCCC has been to implement universal design across the Syracuse University campus. A universal design approach to support the needs of students is an alternative to a "retrofit" approach, as accommodations are built into the environment from the outset, rather than as an afterthought. Having experienced the burden and stigma of the institutional process of disability "retrofit" accommodations, we have advocated for universally designed approaches to learning and instruction at our university (Burgstahler, 2015; Rose & Meyer, 2002). Each fall, leaders of undergraduate student organizations—social and academic groups formed by students—attend our workshops as part of their mandatory trainings. Student organizations don't usually receive any guidance or support to follow ADA regulations, or go beyond such compliance, when planning events. We aimed to make student leaders more aware of the barriers that disabled students face to full participation in campus activities. Additionally, we shared suggestions to make events more inclusive, collaborating with the university's ADA Coordinator in these training sessions to encourage the administration to advance beyond compliance.

When one of us designed a course with flexible policies that incorporated many disability accommodations, we created a video documenting the students' perspectives on the course. Flexible policies were available for all students, regardless of disability, and included extensions on assignments, extended time to complete exams, access to a smaller testing environment, and access to a computer for taking notes in class or for use when completing exams. In the video, several students who did not identify with a disability reported that they felt they were better able to demonstrate their knowledge because of the flexible classroom policies. One student who did identify with a disability and typically requested accommodations, discussed how the flexible policies removed the need to discuss accommodations. Another student said that these policies took away from the stigma of identifying with a disability because supports were offered for all students. We received students' permission to show the videos at public forums to advocate for the use of universal design.

These videos were (and are) used for university wide advocacy. We designed a workshop for incoming teaching assistants (TA) that is presented at an annual TA orientation. Each year, approximately 350 new graduate TAs participate in a three-day orientation. We presented our workshop for faculty and staff members in the School of Education to discuss how to create inclusive college classrooms using Universal Design for Learning principles (Rose & Meyer, 2002). We also co-organized and presented at a forum of faculty and staff from across campus with our university's Office of Disability Services. At these workshops, we introduce a universal design approach to accommodations and share the videos of students who attended classes where flexible policies were applied.

Our advocacy for accessibility urged participants to consider new ways to think and act as members of the university community, in the classroom and in the residence halls. However, students advocating to make their university a place that is accessible and that values disabled people should know that by cooperating with university administrators, their advocacy could inadvertently enable the university to continue its efforts at minimal compliance, which is unlikely to accomplish meaningful access. For example, we worked for hours to create videos that were used in the campus-wide forum about accessibility, but after the forum we learned that the videos were mandated in a resolution following an Office of Civil Rights complaint against the university. While we feel these videos had great impact in presenting practices that are beyond compliance, we were angered by how our labor was used to unknowingly rectify a compliance failure. The lessons we have learned about advocacy center around the relationship between our group and those with decision-making power at the university, specifically the administration. This has forced us to reconsider an approach based on "advocacy."

CHALLENGES WHEN ADVOCATING FOR BEYOND COMPLIANCE AT THE NEOLIBERAL UNIVERSITY

At their base, universities are profit-driven institutions that will accommodate disabled students only insofar as it serves their interests. Institutions are legally required to rectify past wrongs and address disability rights in response to complaints about inequality and discrimination from disabled students, faculty and staff. In doing so, they aim to minimize the possibility of future legal or civil rights complaints against the university. Marketing material that positions an institution as welcoming to a diverse student body can attract a larger number and wider range of prospective students. Marketing the institution as "accessible" and "inclusive" is one way to achieve this and, in turn, can generate more tuition revenue. Disability services formed on U.S. campuses when, following World War I, (mostly white, male) veterans—many of whom were disabled—gained access to higher educational assistance through the 1918 Vocational Rehabilitation Act (Madaus, 2011; Madaus et al., 2009; Mencke, 2010). Universities sought to appear military-friendly to secure guaranteed GI Bill tuition dollars from student veterans. In its origins, then, disability services developed to accommodate the influx of disabled students who brought guaranteed tuition dollars.

As a student advocacy group, we've seen how readily our institution will co-opt rhetoric around accessibility to legitimize further neoliberal goals and ideologies.

For example, the university recently installed heated sidewalks and then touted this as a move to improve accessibility for people with physical disabilities, rather than as a means to avoid paying unionized workers dignified wages to remove snow and ice. Attempts to portray superficial beautification projects as accessibility improvements are also increasingly common across U.S. campuses. In 2016, the university constructed a six million dollar "promenade," which was dishonestly promoted as a project to enhance ADA compliance and promote accessibility, despite blocking off public bus access to central areas of campus and the fact that stairs comprise a significant part of the promenade's design. The announcement of the promenade construction also came shortly after a buyout of more than 250 employees (6.9% of SU's benefits-eligible staff), framed by administration as a necessary cost-cutting measure (Seltzer, 2016).

While the university was spending tens of millions on gymnasium renovations—including a climbing wall and water park—graduate student employees were removed from the employee health insurance plan and forced onto a student plan, one that is far costlier for students with chronic health conditions and other disabilities that require ongoing medical care (Brown, 2018). The gymnasium renovations are part of a larger $255 million campus renovation project being marketed as an investment in and commitment to accessibility and universal design (Carlson, 2017). Using accessibility as a stand-in for corporatization and making cursory nods toward disability diversity does nothing to address the structural issues that render particular body-mind differences disabling.

Beyond the co-optation of rhetoric, we've also learned that universities can be quick to exploit the labor of disabled students to address their own compliance failures. Disabled students are asked to perform unpaid labor to help universities rectify inaccessibility, and then we are expected to be grateful for these opportunities to "be included." Disabled students' participation in university working groups, listening sessions, and open forums—which is rarely compensated—gets used to provide an outward display of inclusivity, but more often than not these groups lack any real decision-making power and fail to yield lasting structural change.

It is the activism and collective organizing of disabled students making public demands on the institution—not the "goodwill" of institutions, or those with institutional power—that has historically resulted in the most significant advances in radical accessibility. For example, at Syracuse University in 2014, a collective of undergraduate and graduate students, faculty, and staff, under the name THE General Body, occupied an administrative building for 18 days. We were protesting cuts to programs for students of color, the sudden closing of the sexual assault Advocacy Center, a lack of mental health support, and architectural and pedagogical inaccessibility. This led, among other changes, to the long overdue hiring of an ADA Coordinator (Mulhere, 2014). THE General Body protest demonstrated the power of collective direct action where advocacy alone failed.

LESSON LEARNED: MOVING FROM ADVOCATE TO ACTIVIST

The terms advocacy and activism may seem synonymous, or at least closely related; activism involves advocating, and advocates often participate in activist movements. Reflecting on our work as disabled students and allies, we have come to understand significant differences between activism and advocacy, and that our group had become too advocacy focused. We saw that this approach, while achieving some progress, had also limited our impact. Seeking change through activism—making collective demands and building public pressure to force their implementation—is a far more fruitful avenue for change than collaboration with those in positions of institutional power.

Advocating for universally designed approaches may achieve awareness, but not the structural and institutional changes needed to make campuses truly accessible to disabled people. Disabled student advocacy can enable administrators to defer costlier structural changes—like the provision of material support for disabled students—with the added benefit to the university that this student labor is unpaid. For example, we took on the role of trying to ensure that students on our campus plan accessible events, implying in some way that access to campus events should be the *responsibility* of students with disabilities. Additionally, we agreed to facilitate a relationship between administrators and blind students, when the university was seeking to address the inaccessibility of a new online platform. This type of advocacy only led to a slow, after-the-fact (retro), effort of minimal compliance and would likely have achieved better results for disabled students if we had collectively boycotted the use of the inaccessible platform.

Instead of advocacy through cooperation, students might deliberately draw attention to their refusal to participate in inaccessible campus events. Only when we refused to participate in a discussion about "promoting accessibility" did we witness the success of the student occupation of an administrative building. Activism, not just advocacy, is necessary for universities to move away from a focus on minimal compliance and superficial references to their accessibility effort. To avoid the co-opting of accessibility by universities and to achieve a community that moves beyond compliance, student organizing toward disability justice—which is anti-racist, anti-imperialist, anti-capitalist, and anti-heterosexist—will continue to be imperative. We cannot expect disability justice to result from advocacy, or working through institutionally-sanctioned channels and processes, alone. Moves toward disability justice result from activism that demands change and applies broad public pressure to get demands met. Enclaves of radical disabled student activists on many campuses are demanding concrete, structural changes to universities that still often fail to meet basic compliance standards.

DEMAND BEYOND COMPLIANCE

Campus initiatives, programs and offices that claim to focus on "diversity" and multiculturalism often fail to address the inequality and exclusion of disabled people resultant from discriminatory practices in higher education (Kim & Aquino, 2017). "Diversity" and "inclusion" offices have different titles and mandates at different institutions. They have countless meetings and set up committees and task groups devoted to diversity and inclusion. Nonetheless, across the U.S. campus movements led by students of color and Indigenous, queer, disabled, and trans* students attest to the inadequacy of administrative lip-service to diversity for challenging systems of oppression and exploitation. These students recognize that universities were never intended for them. Mia Mingus (2017) suggests that "we can do access in liberatory ways that aren't just about inclusion, diversity and equality; but are rather, in service of justice, liberation and interdependence" (Liberatory Access & Interdependence, para. 1). Simple recognition of disability as diversity does not go far enough (Broderick & Lalvani, 2017).

Conversations about disability in higher education traditionally take place around accommodations and services that are "special" and the responsibility of a single office, typically referred to as disability support or disability services offices (DSO). Even though disability legislation—itself the result of disabled people's activism—has prompted universities to accept more disabled students and provide services to them, disability remains absent from the curriculum and institutional culture (Davis, 2011). These initiatives also ignore the role of universities, as corporate entities, in replicating disability injustice locally, nationally, and globally. "Tolerance in its multicultural guise," writes Kelly, drawing on Wendy Brown; "is the liberal answer to managing difference but with no corresponding transformation in the conditions that, in the first place, marked certain bodies as suspicious, deviant, abject, or illegible. Tolerance, therefore, de-politicizes genuine struggles for justice and power" (Kelly, 2016, para 10). Kelley points to student protestors, like those at UNC Chapel Hill, who offer "a model for radical global politics" with demands that

> include ending ties to prisons and sweated labor; retraining and disarming campus police; offering free childcare for students, staff, and faculty; and paying a minimum wage of $25 per hour for workers, with the addendum 'that all administrators be compensated at the same rate as workers' ... unveiling the university's exploitative practices and its deeply embedded structures of racism, sexism, and class inequality can be profound acts of demystification on their own (para 13).

In 2011, the founding members of the BCCC recognized that long term institutional change would only come from disabled students and allies insisting on broader cultural change that affirms the value of disabled lives. Reflecting on our work and the work of student protesters nationally over the last few years, and building off Kelley's insight, we suggest that student movements can do meaningful and necessary activist work to challenge the role universities play in replicating disability oppression and exploitation as it manifests in the local campus context and as it ripples out, affecting communities far beyond the gated walls of predominantly white, corporate universities. We are inspired and energized by the current work of Syracuse University students with the Recognize Us movement, led by disabled and nondisabled women of color, who are refusing superficial nods to access and inclusion and organizing around demands that embody and insist upon an approach that goes beyond compliance.

Note

i ... Trans* includes all transgender, non-binary, and gender nonconforming identities.

REFERENCES

Broderick, A., & Lalvani, P. (2017). Dysconscious ableism: Toward a liberatory praxis in teacher education. *International Journal of Inclusive Education*, *21*(9), 894–905. https://doi.org/10.1080/13603116.2017.1296034

Brown, L. (2018, March 26). Architecture professor responds to plans for Archbold Gymnasium renovations. *The Daily Orange*. Letter to the Editor. Retrieved from http://dailyorange.com/2018/03/architecture-professor-responds-plans-archbold-gymnasium-renovations/

Burgstahler, S. E. (2015). *Universal design in higher education: From principles to practice*. Cambridge, MA: Harvard Education Press.

Carlson, C. (2017, July 20). Six years later, Syracuse's Carrier Dome questions remain unanswered. *The Post-Standard*. Retrieved from http://www.syracuse.com/orangesports/index.ssf/2017/05/six_years_later_question_of_carrier_dome_lingers_at_syracuse_university.html

Cory, R. C., White, J. M., & Stuckey, Z. (2010). Using disability studies theory to change disability services: A case study in student activism. *Journal of Postsecondary Education & Disability*, *23*(1), 28–37.

DaDeppo, L. M. (2009). Integration factors related to the academic success and intent to persist of college students with learning disabilities. *Learning Disabilities Research & Practice*, *24*(3), 122–131.

Davis, L. J. (2011, September 25). Why is disability missing from the discourse on diversity? *The Chronicle of Higher Education*. Retrieved from https://www.chronicle.com/article/Why-Is-Disability-Missing-From/129088

Evans, N. J., Broido, E. M., Brown, K. R., & Wilke, A. K. (2017). *Disability in higher education: A social justice approach*. Hoboken, NJ: John Wiley & Sons.

Kelley, R. D. G. (2016, March 7). Black study, black struggle. *Boston Review*. Retrieved from http://bostonreview.net/forum/robin-d-g-kelley-black-study-black-struggle

Kim, E., & Aquino, K. C. (2017). *Disability as diversity in higher education: Policies and practices to enhance student success*. New York, NY: Taylor & Francis.

Madaus, J. W. (2011, Summer). The history of disability services in higher education. *New Directions for Higher Education, 154*, 5–15.

Madaus, J. W., Miller II, W. K., & Vance, M. L. (2009). Veterans with disabilities in postsecondary education. *Journal of Postsecondary Education and Disability, 22*(1), 10–17. Retrieved from http://files.eric.ed.gov/fulltext/EJ844247.pdf

Meekosha, H., & Shuttleworth, R. (2009). What's so "critical" about critical disability studies? *Australian Journal of Human Rights, 15*(1), 47–75.

Mencke, B. K. B. (2010). *Education, racism, and the military: A critical race theory analysis of the GI Bill and its implications for African Americans in higher education* (Doctoral Dissertation). Retrieved from ProQuest Dissertations Publishing. (Accession No. 3445381).

Mingus, M. (2017, April 12). Access intimacy, interdependence and disability justice. *Leaving Evidence* [blog]. Retrieved from https://leavingevidence.wordpress.com/2017/04/12/access-intimacy-interdependence-and-disability-justice/

Mulhere, K. (2014, November 21). Syracuse U. students end sit-in. *Inside Higher Ed*. Retrieved from https://www.insidehighered.com/quicktakes/2014/11/21/syracuse-u-students-end-sit

Rose, D. H., & Meyer, A. (2002). *Teaching every student in the digital age: Universal design for learning*. Alexandria, VA: Association for Supervision and Curriculum Development.

Seltzer, R. (2016, May 11). Millions for a promenade. *Inside Higher Ed*. Retrieved from https://www.insidehighered.com/news/2016/05/11/syracuse-university-promenade-plan-exposes-tension-between-chancellor-and-faculty

Shallish, L. (2017). A different disability? Challenging the exclusion of disability studies from higher education research and practice. In E. Kim & K. C. Aquino (Eds.), *Disability as diversity in higher education: Policies and practices to enhance student success* (pp. 19–30). New York, NY: Taylor & Francis.

Shildrick, M. (2012). Critical disability studies. In N. Watson, A. Roulstone, & C. Thomas (Eds.), *Routledge Handbook of Disability Studies* (pp. 30–41). New York, NY: Routledge.

Wong, A. (2018, February 14). 6 things can you do to protect disability rights today. *Teen Vogue*. Retrieved from https://www.teenvogue.com/story/disability-rights-how-to-help

CHAPTER 9

Reasonable Adjustments

GEORGE LOW

INTRODUCTION

"Reasonable adjustments" or "reasonable accommodations" describe the steps institutions and organisations must take to avoid prejudice against disabled people. The basic concept remains the same whatever the descriptor; they are measures implemented to help remove barriers to learning that disabled people may experience as a result of their impairments. Among the most obvious examples of reasonable adjustments are the installation of ramps to access buildings, the provision of screen readers for people with sight impairment and installing a hearing loop system for people who have a hearing impairment.

In an ideal world there would be no need for reasonable adjustments, all venues would be accessible to all, all teaching material and methods would be delivered in a way that everyone could understand and engage without any form of adjustment. Since we do not live in an ideal world, the implementation of reasonable adjustments is a useful method of enabling disabled students to attend university, and so they can be an important component of university life for any disabled student.

There are many factors that can have a significant impact on the efficacy of reasonable adjustments, but this chapter will focus on two elements that have a significant impact on the implementation of adjustments; poor communication between staff members causing delays in implementation, and the tendency of universities to categorise impairments into broad classes such as mobility impairment or sight impairment instead of considering the unique impact of impairments on individuals (Low, 2018). These are key factors in what will become clear in this chapter: reasonable adjustments can form an essential component in a disabled student's journey through the education system. However, they often fail to meet their objective.

Reasonable adjustments are not implemented as efficiently as they should be, despite the duty to undertake them, their implementation can be haphazard, and they can vary depending on the individual tasked to carry them out (Riddell & Weedon, 2014). This chapter will highlight some of those limitations and suggest strategies to improve the efficacy of reasonable adjustments for the benefit of students and to ensure that the best strategies and practices are in place so that lecturers and support staff have the knowledge and means to provide efficient support for disabled students which in turn will help universities comply with any regulations.

THE PHYSICAL ASPECT OF REASONABLE ADJUSTMENTS

The most obvious factor that can influence the efficacy of reasonable adjustments is the physical environment such as the design or construction of a building, any approach to, exit from, or access to a building, fixtures, fittings, furnishings, furniture, equipment or other moveable property in or on premises. From a wheelchair user's perspective, ramps, lifts (elevators), doorways, room sizes and the availability of accessible toilets all impact on their ability to move around campus. These are obvious areas where reasonable adjustments can prove effective in providing access to what would otherwise be inaccessible venues.

It is reasonable to assume that most universities in developed nations will attempt to meet their legal obligations under specific legislation, such as the UK Equality Act (2010) and the US Americans with Disabilities Act (1990) to make their campuses accessible. The nature of many university campuses can make this difficult however as some, especially in Europe, have very old buildings that present major challenges. Ramps, stair-lifts, and automatic doors are the standard method of providing better access, but there are various challenges that must be negotiated when retrospectively installing means of access. Technical difficulties, such as finding a suitable location to install a lift (elevator) or finding the space to install a ramp, must be considered along with the restrictions imposed by local building regulations and preservation orders.

Universities around the world have many challenges to negotiate when attempting to make campuses fully accessible. While efforts are made by universities to meet the requirements of disabled students, these efforts are often hampered by the challenges related to the age of buildings and health and safety regulations, meaning many of the provisions made to improved access are compromised or negated. Governments enact laws such as the Equality Act 2010 (UK) and the Disability Discrimination Act 1992 (Australia) to help prevent discrimination by penalising institutions that contravene these laws; failure to install a ramp or move a class to an accessible venue is blatant discrimination and consequently a contravention of these laws. So, to avoid putting their disabled students at a disadvantage and breaking any laws, it is in the interest of universities to anticipate issues that may put a student at a disadvantage. In doing so, universities will avoid the possibility of inadvertently discriminating against students while the process of putting appropriate measures in place is underway.

THE DUTY OF UNIVERSITIES TO ANTICIPATE REASONABLE ADJUSTMENTS

In the UK, institutions and organisations have a duty to *anticipate* reasonable adjustments, they should not simply react to the requirements of a new student but should anticipate any adjustments that might be required by any disabled student (The Equality Act (2010) section 20, p. 10). Similar guidelines can be found in other counties around the world (Waddington & Lawson, 2009). Anticipating the requirements of disabled students is important if a university wishes to avoid any form of discrimination against its students. An example of anticipating a reasonable adjustment is the practice of installing hearing loop technology in lecture halls and seminar rooms. In this case, the university is anticipating students with a hearing impairment attending lectures, but often universities will take a reactive rather than proactive approach to reasonable adjustments and only implement measures when an issue is brought to their attention.

A good example of the problems this failure to anticipate reasonable adjustments can have is demonstrated in one of my own experiences as a disabled student. During my PhD course, I was lucky enough to be allocated my current assistance dog, Fogle. Having Fogle with me most of the time meant I would need a toilet facility for him while on campus, so I asked a senior member of staff why there was no dog toilet facility presently available on campus. I was informed that, given the variety and range of severity that exists in relation to impairments, it is not possible for the university to anticipate every disabled student's needs. To quote that member of staff: "The university can provide some adjustments and facilities for its students, but it is up to each student to ask for less common adjustments and facilities" (Low, 2018, p. 227). This policy not only breaks UK law as it is the duty of universities to anticipate adjustments for all students (The Equality Act (2010) section 20, p. 10), but is also employing an approach that implies a hierarchy of impairment by anticipating adjustments for students with more common requirements and not anticipating any measures that may be required for students who need less common adjustments. The university could be perceived as prioritising one type of impairment over another. This approach implies a hierarchy of disability—that the more commonly recognised impairments, and consequently some disabled students, are worthy of more consideration than others.

On a more practical level, not anticipating an adjustment results in a period where the student experiences discrimination until the adjustment is implemented. The experience I had when asking for a toileting facility for Fogle is a good example of this; there was a period of two weeks when I could not attend campus because there was no toilet in place for Fogle who had undergone intense training to ensure he would only use a designated toileting area. Eventually after several changes of location, a toilet was installed in a suitable area and I could return to campus.

PROVIDING AN ADAPTABLE CURRICULUM

The influence of university staff in providing the appropriate measures was caused by two things; the difficulty in understanding the nature of the adjustment required by the member of staff tasked with its implementation, and senior staff's interpretation of the university's duty regarding the anticipation of reasonable adjustments. Along with physical considerations, the influence of staff members play a major role in the implementation of reasonable adjustments and consequently, the efficacy and provision of adjustments can vary depending on the knowledge and training of the people tasked with their implementation. Although the physical aspect of attending a university campus can present challenges for disabled students, issues created by the knowledge and working practices of university staff present a more significant barrier. Poor understanding of the adjustment required, and the interpretation of the university's duties are instrumental in creating difficulties in the provision of reasonable adjustments.

Both elements can be attributed to the decisions and knowledge of the staff; even with the best intentions, things can go wrong if staff are unfamiliar with what is required to put an adjustment in place or if they are not conversant with the university's obligations. This also applies to the way teaching is delivered; courses and curricula are devised and maintained by staff and if these staff members are not familiar with the university's obligations regarding reasonable adjustments, disabled students may experience difficulty in attending a course or managing their studies. An example of this was presented in recent research where a disabled student described the lack of flexibility in the university's curriculum as a barrier; "I've tried to get permission to do my teaching placement part-time and after ... very close to court action really, [they] didn't quite sort of follow through on it actually being part-time" (Low, 2018, pp. 189–190). This shows that a good understanding of the difficulties disabled students can face as they attempt to complete a university qualification is essential if barriers to education are to be removed. University curricula are organised and managed by staff members and if those staff members do not understand the impact that course structures and timetables can have on disabled students, the university will leave itself open to the criticism that they are not providing an equal and inclusive qualification programme. Many factors can impact on disabled students experience as they attend university courses, but an almost hidden symptom that can be overlooked when considering the structure and management of curricula is chronic fatigue.

For disabled students who are enrolled in courses requiring them to attend lectures, seminars or tutorials on a regular basis, fatigue can be an important factor for consideration. Many disabled people have impairments that can impact on their endurance and for some, the impact of chronic fatigue is a symptom that is difficult to convey to others (Low, 2018). Chronic fatigue requires adjustments that allow the student to study at their own pace and for periods of time that would not exacerbate levels of fatigue and this type of flexibility is not easy to find in university teaching methods (Low, 2018). The solution, of course, is to provide a flexible schedule that would take levels of fatigue into consideration. Many of the issues that face disabled students as they attend university can be lessened or avoided if universities provide flexible teaching and curricula. Difficulties experienced on campus can be negated through distance learning which minimises the necessity to spend time on campuses that are not fully suitable for wheelchair users or students with other impairments.

For those courses that cannot be delivered through distance learning, a flexible and adaptable programme can reduce the risk of chronic fatigue impacting on the capacity of disabled students to attend lectures and other course requirements. A curriculum that is flexible enough to allow disabled students the ability to study at a pace and over a timeframe that suits them, would help provide access to learning opportunities for people who have chronic fatigue, difficulties with concentration over a long period, or have chronic pain. Organising and managing such a curriculum would require at least a basic knowledge of disability and the effects of impairments, so any staff member tasked with timetabling or making up course content would benefit from some form of training to ensure they structure the courses and curricula appropriately. It is in these circumstances that issues related to the knowledge and experience of university staff can have a significant impact on the learning experiences of disabled students.

COMMUNICATING AND COLLABORATING WITH STUDENTS

Training staff is just one part of the solution; another way to ensure the requirements of disabled students are well understood is to ensure each student is consulted regularly to ensure their requirements are being met in an efficient manner. Consulting with students is a procedure that most universities carry out in a haphazard manner Riddell and Weedon (2014). There is room for improvement. A "one shoe fits all" approach to reasonable adjustments is a major factor in creating problems, a factor that can be avoided if staff are more familiar with the requirements of individual students. With each impairment is a different set of needs (Shakespeare & Watson, 2002) and measures to alleviate difficulties arising from these individual circumstances can only be effective if there is a good level of knowledge exchange between the provider and recipient. Direct contact between the staff tasked to provide adjustments and the student in question is one way to achieve this.

The most common procedure to ascertain and manage disabled students' requirements is to instruct new students to contact the Student Disability Service (or equivalent support departments) who will generate a schedule of adjustments that should be put in place for that student. This schedule can be monitored through annual reviews by the support service who can ask the student if their circumstances have changed and if their needs are being met. For many students, the only time they will speak in person about their requirements with a member of staff who specialises in the provision of reasonable adjustments is once a year, during their initial meeting. A lot can happen in a year that might impact on the requirements of a disabled person and their access to learning. Students impairments can change, the university's teaching facilities change either through new buildings or the deterioration of older ones, or new technologies can emerge that will make adjustments easier for a university to implement. It is important then that university staff are familiar with the current circumstances of their disabled students.

Meanwhile, disabled students are expected to take the initiative and to report any issues with their adjustments themselves. Circumstances can change significantly for many within a year, and annual monitoring cannot facilitate the communication necessary to ensure adjustments are effective. It is common for disabled people to be stigmatised and regarded as different from non-disabled people and this can impact on their self-esteem and confidence making them reticent in communicating what some others might see as their shortcomings (Goffman, 1963; Nussbaum, 2004; Shakespeare, 1996; Swain & French, 2000). Volunteering what can be very personal information to someone you have not met is not an ideal situation for anyone and this "routine of social intercourse" (Goffman, 1963, p. 12) can be a stressful experience for disabled people who can often resort to downplaying or hiding their impairment to avoid being regarded as "less than" (Darling, 2003, pp. 881–895; Goffman 1963, pp. 41–42; Shakespeare, 1996, p. 7).

The solution is to have a *trained* person available to students who could act as a "go to" when they require support. This will effectively reduce the layers of bureaucracy, complications and delays that can arise when too many individuals are involved in the provision of reasonable adjustments. A "go to" person would give the student direct access to a specific individual who could become familiar with their requirements and give the university a better opportunity to provide adjustments that are tailored to individual students. If the "go to" person was given appropriate authority, they could serve as a conduit that gives the disabled student better and more direct communication with the people who have the power to make changes. They would also provide a more direct and timelier route to the adjustments they need. This strategy could also be strengthened by drawing on the people who are already tasked with supporting students such as student union officials, and disability services departments. One way of doing this would be to have union officials assigned to student disability departments or a union office next to the student disability office. This "student advocacy office" would ensure the disabled student's support person was acting on the interests of the student and was not influenced by the agenda of the university. Each school in the university would have a "go to" person who could be approached by students and that person would have direct access to the "student advocacy office," so students would no longer experience delays and miscommunication as cases are referred through a long series of departments and staff members.

CONCLUSION

Reasonable adjustments are a crucial element of student life that can only be effective if specific practices are put in place. For adjustments to be effective the student has an important part to play. Measures that are tailored to meet the requirements of individual students cannot be implemented without detailed and up to date information from the student in question. It is a false dichotomy to think that reasonable adjustments can be viewed from two perspectives: that of the university whose responsibility it is to ensure the adjustments are effective, and the student for whom the adjustments are implemented. The university staff should have sufficient knowledge of the requirements of each individual student and the measures required to meet those requirements. This can only be achieved through constant and effective communication with the student.

A student advocacy service would serve to address communication issues and disentangle the interests of the student from the difficulties universities can have with the implementation of reasonable adjustments. The difficulties that can arise with interpersonal interaction could also be minimised if the student had regular contact with a disabled student's advocate and their office to build up a strong and beneficial relationship. As I have shown, university staff are not in the best position to ensure disabled students' requirements are met by reasonable adjustments due to the pressures of work and the influence of university agendas. The best way to ensure the efficient implementation of adjustments is to provide a support system independent of the university and advocates with the disabled student's best interest at heart.

REFERENCES

Americans With Disabilities Act of 1990, Pub. L. No. 101–336, 104 Stat. 328 (1990).
Darling, R. B. (2003). Toward a model of changing disability identities: A proposed typology and research agenda. *Disability & Society, 18*(7), 881–895.
Disability Discrimination Act (1990). (ACT) 135, (Australia).
Equality Act 2010 Ch. 15 (UK).
Goffman, E. (1963). *Stigma: Notes on the management of spoiled identity.* London, UK: Penguin.
Low, G. A. (2018). *Where are all the disabled musicians? An exploration of the attitudinal and physical barriers that impact on the identities and lived experiences of musicians with a physical impairment* (Unpublished PhD Thesis). University of Edinburgh, Edinburgh, Scotland.
Nussbaum, M. (2004). *Hiding from humanity: Disgust, shame and the law.* Princeton, NJ: Princeton University Press.
Riddell, S., & Weedon, E. (2014). Changing legislation and its effects on inclusive and special education: Scotland. *British Journal of Special Education, 41*(4), 363–381.
Shakespeare, T. (1996). Disability, identity and difference. In C. Barnes & G. Mercer (Eds.), *Exploring the divide* (pp. 94–113). Leeds, UK: The Disability Press.
Shakespeare, T., & Watson, N. (2002). The social model of disability: An outdated ideology? *Research in Social Science and Disability, 2,* 9–28.
Swain, J., & French, S. (2000). Towards an affirmation model of disability. *Disability & Society, 15*(4), 569–582.
Waddington, L., & Lawson, A. (2009). *Disability and non-discrimination law in the European Union: An analysis of disability discrimination law within and beyond the employment field.* Luxembourg: Publications office of the European Union.

CHAPTER 10

But You Look Fine: Limitations of the Letter of Accommodation

ZOIE SHEETS

TO WHOM IT MAY CONCERN

In my first two years as a student, I received no accommodations and I was intentional about who I disclosed my disability to. My illness is what is often referred to as "contested"; its validity is questioned by many, including those in the medical community. After years of being chronically ill, I was all too familiar with the reactions that would meet me when I chose to disclose to my university. My desire to avoid the pain associated with someone completely dismissing my lived experience kept me from seeking accommodations. However, as my junior year swung into full gear, and the Chicago winter grew colder, my body was sent into an excruciating flare. Standing was a challenge; attending classes was nearly out of the question.

  As I laid on the couch in my dorm room sobbing at the thought of how behind I had fallen and how far my grades would drop, a friend looked at me and said, "You *have* to visit the disability office." A week later, I left my appointment at the Disability Resource Center pleasantly surprised and reassured, armed with a letter of accommodation (LOA). The choice of the word "armed" is intentional. This letter of accommodation would become my only weapon in an intense battle for the accommodations I needed to succeed in my college education. When first presenting my LOA to professors, their eyebrows would often furrow as they looked me up and down. Their looks communicated something like, "But you look fine," often followed with verbal responses indicating the professors' disbelief that they would need to accommodate someone who appeared young and healthy.

The LOA presents a way of fighting against both intentional and unintentional barriers, such as remaining in long courses with no breaks or exams that were too long for my body to sit through. There is a great deal of misunderstanding around the LOA, what it is, why it is used and how it can create opportunities for student success. For example, when a professor admitted, via e-mail, that he wrote a "significantly harder exam for me because students with extra time have an advantage and the playing field should be even," my LOA was the launch pad for a conversation about why accommodations exist.

This chapter continues that conversation. It recognizes that a letter of accommodation can play a role in student success, but that it also has limitations. Speaking both to students and professors, this chapter examines some of the complexities that accompany LOAs, and how creating accessible classrooms *must* extend beyond reliance on their existence.

THE LIMITATIONS OF A LETTER OF ACCOMMODATION

A letter of accommodation (LOA) is a formal document, typically written by a disability services office, requesting accommodations and support for a student with a disability, without altering the course goals (Masinter, 2015). Other higher education institutions will have a similar formal procedure; however, it may have a different title. The letter can serve as a tool for students fighting for their rights to access classrooms fully, however, it can also bring with it a good deal of misunderstanding. Even for the most well-meaning educators, the LOA model can sometimes lead to barriers in the classroom. In the final semester of my undergraduate education, I was told by a professor I could not sit in a chair to present my final project because that "wasn't a need listed in the letter." He emphasized how important it would be for me to be able to present standing in my future career, so I stood through the presentation I had worked for months on as my pain levels continued to rise and my legs began to tremble. As will be expanded on later, considering a LOA alone as sufficient for creating an accessible classroom can leave some access needs unmet (Evans et al., 2017).

LOAs can fall short in other ways as well. First, accommodations are different from accessibility (Trammell, 2009). Accommodations are changes made to meet individual needs, while an accessible space is constructed in a way that accommodations don't have to be as heavily relied upon. Access is preferred to accommodation, because accommodation shifts the burden to disabled students and forces disclosure, which can be risky. Disabled identities are, unfortunately, still stigmatized, particularly in academic settings which emphasize accommodations over broadened access. This means that disclosing a disabled identity, especially for contested illnesses, can invite alienation, stigmatization, and marginalization (Trammell, 2009). The stigma encountered by disabled students can make it hard to become fully immersed in academic communities and in social opportunities (Trammell, 2009). Additionally, the disclosure required by an LOA-only model can have a lasting impact on student-professor relationships.

An accessible classroom considers the incredible diversity of the minds and bodies that may enter the room, and makes proactive changes to promote positive learning outcomes (Chandler et al., 2017). While accommodations can play a key role in creating accessible classrooms, educators must also understand that LOAs alone will not make a classroom fully accessible for students to understand material and demonstrate their knowledge. In addition to the limitations mentioned above, LOAs cannot adequately address the unpredictable nature of some disabilities, including chronic illness. Access needs are dynamic and can shift quickly, much more quickly than a university's disability office can rewrite a letter.

Pointing out limitations of letters of accommodation does not undermine their importance. Rather, the solution to ensure students with disabilities can fully participate in classrooms is two-fold. Both students and educators must understand how to navigate using an LOA, and the idea of what accessibility in a classroom looks like in practice must be expanded. Below are discussions of both the student and professor perspective of navigating the "accommodations talk"—the moment a LOA is first presented. This initial conversation plays an important role in the implementation of a LOA, as well as a discussion of moving beyond an LOA-only model.

DEAR STUDENTS: YOUR LETTER OF ACCOMMODATIONS

The "accommodations talk" is challenging. There are many reactions that may follow placing the letter in front of an educator. Negative reactions, such as pity or doubt, have the potential to negatively impact every day spent in that particular classroom. Unfortunately, there is no formula to ensure the perfect or most supportive reaction. There are, however, a few steps that can be taken to make the experience, and the many days of the semester that follow, the best possible. It is important to recognize that the labor of making a classroom accessible should not fall on the shoulders of disabled students, but that self-advocacy and communication are also deeply-rooted parts of the disability experience and culture. If, even after using these suggestions, the reaction of an educator is harmful, students should know who to go to on campus for the support needed. For example, if a professor were to refuse to accommodate a student for any reason, question a student's disability status, or question a student's belonging in the class, a student should be aware what office or campus entity they can visit for support.

When first presenting a LOA to a professor, a student should request an in-person meeting with them. It is important that presenting a letter of accommodation be a conversation, including follow-up questions, clarifications, and more. While it is arguably much easier to e-mail a LOA, or hand it in while entering class on the first day, sitting down to talk can increase the chances that the LOA will be used appropriately. Sometimes conversations about LOAs can be filled with many questions. The questions are an opportunity for an educator to learn more. The student is the expert of their own experience, their own disability, and their own access needs. Both the educator and student should trust and respect this expertise. Professors cannot ask about a specific diagnosis, and a student can decline to answer questions that cause discomfort (Evans et al., 2017).

Sometimes LOAs have only one or two accommodations listed, but if a student experiences anything like I do, the letter may have many more. Each accommodation may apply differently from classroom to classroom, or from activity to activity. For example, if there is extended time on evaluations, this time may be needed for long exams that are taxing on the body, but not for short 10-minute quizzes. The conversation should be guided from accommodation to accommodation so that both student and professor know exactly what each accommodation will look like in that classroom.

If there is a specific part of the class a student is concerned about accessing, this needs to be communicated. No professor, whether they are disabled or not, trained in access or not, will ever be able to predict every access need. This meeting is the place to explore ways to make even the most challenging aspects of a class accessible. Any disability-friendly learning space must be flexible (Neill & Etheridge, 2008). Access needs change, particularly when disabilities evolve or are episodic. It can be helpful to explicitly remind an educator that if another access need arises, or a part of the class isn't fully accessible to the student, there will need to be a follow-up.

DEAR PROFESSOR: RESPONDING TO LETTERS OF ACCOMMODATIONS

Creating accessible spaces is challenging. It requires creativity, communication, and commitment. It is important to recognize this challenge, and equally important to recognize that it is a challenge that is not optional to undertake. All students deserve a space that is accessible to their body and mind. The impact of education on lifetime wellbeing is far too great for us to exclude any students from learning, whether it is intentional or not.

On my campus, I have been involved in disability advocacy and I have had countless conversations with professors and administrators. Through these conversations, I have noticed that a majority of professors have shared that they either had an understanding that accessibility was important but didn't have the knowledge and skills to create it, or that they hadn't necessarily considered accessibility a vital part of their classroom. Essentially, there was a lack of knowledge about disability culture and experience, and the ways they inform classroom experience. Professors are not always provided with the resources they need to create classrooms fully welcoming of disabled students and may, as a result, go years without examining the consequences of their actions. This can even cause them to feel defensive when they are eventually asked to do so. In follow-up conversations, professors often reveal their defensiveness was rooted in frustration. Why hadn't someone shared these ideas sooner? Sharing ideas, lessons learned, and feedback is critical to creating an accessible classroom. While letters of accommodations are included in the umbrella of "accessible classroom," this idea must extend further than LOAs because of the limitations of an accommodations-based model (Evans et al., 2017; Trammell, 2009).

It is illegal in the United States and many other countries to ask students the specifics of their impairments (Evans et al., 2017). Since students have varying levels of comfort with their disability, some may choose to disclose more than others, but that has to be a decision made by the individual. Knowing a diagnosis doesn't prepare an educator to create a better classroom environment. Instead, listening to a student talk about how their disability interacts with their classroom experience prepares an educator to do this. Responding to letters of accommodation is not optional; when a student has an LOA, a professor must provide accommodations (Evans et al., 2017). The "accommodations talk" serves as a launch pad for the process of creating an accessible classroom, and there are several steps that can be taken to ensure the process is beneficial for both educator and student.

Students with disabilities have often had to fight hard to receive their accommodations and simply exist in spaces, particularly higher education spaces. Higher education spaces are often constructed in ways that are not accessible, both physically and culturally. If a student seems skeptical of teacher support, or defensive when asked questions, there is typically a reason for this. Don't meet their skepticism with frustration, but rather continually remind them that it is the job of the educator to support their learning. Listen actively. Students with disabilities have often not had ideal experiences in higher education (Jacklin et al., 2007). Listening actively, making eye contact and showing understanding can help a student know that their professor is invested in making the classroom a space they can succeed in. Asking questions is an integral part of active listening, and also gives the professor a chance to make sure they fully understand the accommodations asked for in the LOA. If there are any questions about how to make the classroom work for the student, always ask so that the situation can be proactively addressed.

The student is the expert of their own situation, disabilities, and needs. No matter how many classes a professor has taught, or how many students with disabilities they have worked with, the particular student in front of them knows their disability better than anyone in the world. In addition, there will be students with multiple disabilities, so the access needs on their letter of accommodation can vary from what may be previously understood about a student's disability status. There are many myths about letters of accommodation that can harm students. Knowing these myths can help avoid perpetuating them. One such "myth" is that letters of accommodations make it easier for students with disabilities to succeed by giving them a "running start," or putting them ahead of the starting line. In fact, LOAs act to level the playing field by lessening the barriers that disabled students face (Hodge & Preston-Sabin, 1997). Another myth is the idea of "overcoming." Many people with disabilities view their disability as something powerful, something to be proud of, and a part of their identity. Their desire is not to overcome, but to exist in spaces that recognizes their wholeness, their needs, and their contributions (Brown, 2003). Even if a student is not at a point where they feel this way toward their disability, a professor's responsibility is not to push a student toward overcoming—it's to make sure there aren't barriers in the classroom that need to be overcome in the first place.

CREATING ACCESSIBLE CLASSROOMS

While responding to LOAs in an intentional and supportive manner is a key component of creating accessible classrooms, it is not the only component. Accessibility goes much deeper than accommodations (Trammell, 2009). Accommodations respond to individual needs, where an accessible space is an environment that, *from the beginning*, is constructed in a manner that allows all minds and bodies to fully participate (Evans et al., 2017). Moving toward accessibility not only mitigates some of the limitations of a LOA, such as the risks of disclosure, but has various other benefits, including creating new ways for both disabled and non-disabled students to engage with materials, challenging instructors to develop innovative teaching methods, and saving the time typically dedicated to creating separate accommodations for each individual student (Evans et al., 2017). While self-advocacy and communication will continue to hold a crucial role in the disabled student experience, the burden of access labor is transitioned to the educators. Many disability resource practitioners argue this expansion beyond legally-required accommodations is key to student success (Evans et al.,

2017). Piecing together accommodations on a situational basis simply doesn't lead to complete, social and academic participation (Satz, 2008).

Creating an accessible classroom entails recognizing various forms of access, including physical, sensory, cognitive, and linguistic. The concept of universal design was created to describe ways to make the built environment fully accessible to all bodies, and the idea of an accessible classroom extends this to learning (Chandler et al., 2017). It considers not only the physical classroom, but teaching methods, testing and presentation requirements, language use, and more, with the intention of maximizing learning outcomes without lowering expectations (Chandler et al., 2017). Often, when considering accessibility, ramps immediately come to mind, but access goes much deeper than that. In a classroom setting, physical access may also include having a policy that allows students to come and go from a classroom in case anxiety, pain, or fatigue levels spike. Sensory access can include showing videos with captions, ensuring documents are equipped with text recognition capabilities, and verbally describing any information that is communicated visually. Pausing between asking a question and calling on a student can provide cognitive access by allowing students' thoughts to catch up with the lecture, and sensory access aides such as ASL interpreters or captionists to catch up as well. There are a wide array of things to consider when creating accessible classrooms, many of which will not be explicitly listed in a LOA.

Finally, a letter of accommodation will not include information on classroom climate, which is also vital for an accessible classroom. A study conducted at Baylor University found that, while accommodations can be necessary at times, they are only effective if provided by a caring staff that aim to build a trusting relationship and empower students (Graham-Smith & Lafayette, 2004). Faculty attitudes directly impact not only their relationship with disabled students, but also the way other students react to disabled peers in the classroom. The Baylor study also identified that many of the stresses impacting disabled students were either caused or exacerbated by staff and faculty that had inadequate knowledge of access, or lack of intent in creating access. Expanding beyond a letter-of-accommodation model to aim for classroom accessibility can challenge able-bodied staff, faculty, and students' perception of disability, creating an environment more welcoming of disabled students and supportive of their success.

Disability is diverse, intersectional, and fluid. No one will ever understand every access need and how to address it; however, we can challenge ourselves to continue learning and expanding our understanding collaboratively. Since disability is such a varied experience, a letter of accommodation can simply not capture all that is needed to make a classroom accessible. LOAs are based in legal compliance, limiting their capacity to acknowledge the role of disability culture and identity in the classroom. Beginning with the "accommodations talk," semester-long communication between professors and disabled students can contribute to student success. In higher education systems, there is not yet enough shared knowledge or resources to ensure every classroom is fully accessible. It is imperative that this goal is not forgotten. In the meantime, however, using this twofold approach—recognizing LOAs can be part of access but are not the whole of it—can fill many of the gaps impacting disabled students' academic success and enjoyment.

REFERENCES

Brown, S. E. (2003). *Movie stars and sensuous scars: Essays on the journey from disability shame to disability pride.* New York, NY: iUniverse.

Chandler, R., Zaloudek, J. A., & Carlson, K. (2017). How do you intentionally design to maximize success in the academically diverse classroom? *New Directions for Teaching and Learning, 2017*(151), 151–169.

Evans, N. J., Broido, E. M., Brown, K. R., & Wilke, A. K. (2017). *Disability in higher education: A social justice approach.* San Francisco, CA: Jossey-Bass.

Graham-Smith, S., & Lafayette, S. (2004). Quality disability support for promoting belonging and academic success within the college community. *College Student Journal, 38*(1), 90.

Hodge, B. M., & Preston-Sabin, J. (Eds.). (1997). *Accommodations—or just good teaching? Strategies for teaching college students with disabilities.* Westport, CT: Praeger.

Jacklin, A., Robinson, C., O'Meara, L., & Harris, A. (2007). *Improving the experiences of disabled students in higher education.* Brighton, UK: The Higher Education Academy. Retrieved from http://cascadeoer2.pbworks.com/w/file/fetch/33757279/jacklin.pdf

Masinter, M. R. (2015). Avoid the word "reasonable" in accommodations policy. *Disability Compliance for Higher Education, 21*(3), 3.

Neill, S., & Etheridge, R. (2008). Flexible learning spaces: The integration of pedagogy, physical design, and instructional technology. *Marketing Education Review, 18*(1), 47–53.

Satz, A. B. (2008). Disability, vulnerability, and the limits of antidiscrimination. *Washington Law Review, 83*, 513.

Trammell, J. (2009). Red-shirting college students with disabilities. *Learning Assistance Review, 14*(2), 21–31.

CHAPTER 11

The Need for Systemic Supports: Barriers Faced by Students with Disabilities in the Majority World

MOSTAFA ATTIA

Arab societies always treated certain categories of disabled persons as a negligible quantity, treating them as though it was the end of the road. Disability in Arab culture has traditionally been seen as something shameful, an ordeal to be endured by the family. (Nagata, 2007, unpaged)

INTRODUCTION

Disability rights have come to the forefront of many global policies and debates over recent years. The wider ratification of the UNCRPD starting form 2006, as well as the emergence of post-2015 new global discourses (SDGs), emphasize the importance of creating inclusive educational environments through applying the required accommodations. While the reasonable accommodation procedures are clearly outlined by the treaty, wide variation of implementation of these regulations is reported throughout the literature (IDA, 2016). Meeting these regulations demands more consistency in practice.

Egypt, (the case study of this section) has ratified both the UNCRPD in 2008 as well as signing the SDGs in 2015, with a mass revolution in between. Its slogan "bread, freedom and social justice," paved the way for marginalised groups to raise their voices up along with others. (Mittermaier, 2014) This elucidation of a participatory approach may enforce listening to the voices and demands of students with disabilities. Undoubtedly, disabled people were among the Egyptians who benefitted from these developments, at least at the policy level. Their participation in the Egyptian constitution issued in 2014 included 8 subjects with reference to the rights of disabled people, among which were education and higher education policies. (Constitute Project, 2014. See for example articles 53, 81, 214 and 244 of Egypt's Constitution of 2014.) Most recently, the new disability Law issued in 2018 addressed the necessity for disabled students to be mainstreamed in both education and higher education with reasonable accommodation in place. (New Law for Persons with Disabilities, 2018.) It could be argued that the results of these policies could be seen in both disabled people organizations (DPOs) initiatives as well as an outpouring of funds from the international organizations to equip the university with reasonable accommodation measures to support the inclusivity of higher education.

This chapter contextualizes the barriers facing majority world students with disabilities in higher education. These challenges start from the admission process through to the different stages of university academic life. This chapter critiques what is missing in student support and gives recommendations to higher education institutions of what they should have in place. While this chapter may concentrate more specifically on institutions in Egypt, it will remain useful and relevant to an international audience, especially from other majority world countries.

Student advocacy and demands for necessary supports will influence university senior management to formulate a diversity and equality strategy aiming to develop an inclusive environment. This chapter will focus on admissions procedures, which are frequently influenced and determined by a person's impairment, rather than their qualifications. This discussion will also include course of study submission arrangements and exam procedures. Through this exposure, the student will similarly be given insight into what they should expect from the university they attend.

While in the global north countries there has been considerable progress regarding provisions made for students with disabilities, Arab countries may require more research in the field of higher education. Egyptian universities lack systematic support that they can offer to students with disabilities during their academic life, and as a result, support is ad-hoc in nature. While positive examples include braille centres and providing some mobility and orientation training to familiarise students with disabilities with the campus environment, its arbitrary nature aggravates problems confronted with admissions, during the course of study and exam periods. This necessitates, as this chapter argues, the development of a more systemic approach to supporting students with disabilities.

ADMISSIONS

According to the Egyptian Supreme Council of Universities established in 1950, universities can accept students with disabilities who are either blind or physically impaired as long as they achieved a 50% (pass) at their secondary school (TEMPUS, undated). The majority of people with other impairments, however, are deprived from accessing higher education. The policies and legislation regarding the admission of students with disabilities into universities, and their rights once at university, are inadequate (Egyptian Ministry of Higher Education, 1972). Although little research exists around the situation in developing countries, the barriers preventing students with disabilities accessing higher education in the Egyptian context could be similar to those in other countries (Salmi & Bassett, 2012). Support is geared towards three types of disability: blindness, deafness and physical disability. Most institutions cater for students who are either blind or use a wheel chair. Many institutions excuse their lack of support through the non-existence of funding (Matshedisho, 2007).

The treatment of the non-disabled population is very different in terms of university admission structure. The arbitrary nature of the acceptance criteria at both faculty and department levels leaves the admission decision in the hands of the faculty deans, relying solely on their understanding and knowledge when accepting or rejecting disabled applicants. As a disabled researcher insider, I am aware of many disabled colleagues who were refused entry to a specific department in one university, while others were accepted the year after. I faced a similar experience when applying to an institution. Although I stated full responsibility for my disability requirements, the Dean was opposed to a blind person entering the school, assuming that the latter would not have the necessary equipment to accommodate my needs. While many of the newly-emerged disability rights based policies were issued following the Egyptian revolution in 2011, the question is to what extent this actually influences university staff awareness and effects the admission process equally for students with disabilities. There are still many obstacles faced by the disabled when applying to university, including clear information about where to go or to whom they can direct their questions (USAID, 2017).

Typical of many other students, due to the inaccessibility of the admissions process, I relied mostly on friends who volunteered to fill out my application forms. All letters and confirmation documents that I received were not in an accessible format. Although the university employees were very helpful in assisting me through the whole admissions process, this support was based on their *willingness* to help instead of following a structured plan coming from an organized system. This may include providing a basic training to the university admissions staff on how they can best support individuals with different impairments. Improving the system may have to rely on students with disabilities' experiences throughout the admissions process, turning the difficulties that they faced into lessons learned.

The development of university orientation procedures for students with disabilities is another important related issue, especially in their initial weeks (Goode, 2007). It will undoubtedly take longer for students with disabilities to familiarize themselves with the university environment, including lecture venues. Their reliance on their friends for guidance and/or mobility support could cause accidents or injuries due to the former's lack of training.

The admission policy procedures at all universities need to include clear guidelines to ensure the application of accessibility measures, and include students with different types of impairments. This involves preparing the Universities and Faculties admission forms in accessible formats and/or providing Personal Assistants (PA) to assist in these regards. Additionally, the Department's acceptance procedures need to rely on clearer criteria, based on students' qualifications, not his/her impairments. The document outlining this procedure must not only be known by all admissions personnel, it must also be made available to every applicant. These processes must ensure that fair and equitable admissions are available at every university.

The university administration staff should be trained on mobility orientation and how they might assist students with disabilities when they first arrive. This essential training can ideally be facilitated by faculty or students with disabilities themselves—those who know, through their lived experience, what administrative staff need to know. Finally, registering all students with an impairment as disabled may assist university departments in providing the necessary reasonable accommodation, if this registration is coupled with an unwavering commitment to student rights to access and equitable treatment.

DURING THE COURSE OF STUDY

The Egyptian ratification of the UNCRPD, followed by The Egyptian revolution, brought new national discourses to protect the rights of all disabled people, including in the field of higher education. The 2014 Egyptian constitution, followed by the new disability law issued in 2018, could be seen as an advanced legal framework to protect the rights of disabled people. Despite these policy developments, students with disabilities continue to experience difficulty accessing needed support, and as a result, their study (attending lectures, interacting with course materials, communicating with module conveners, and submitting assignments) continues to be fraught with difficulty.

Because of the absence of legal rules regulating academic assistance, there is no consistency in student experience (Attia, 2009). Individual professors' responses to student need differs from course to course, university to university. Relying on faculty or staff willingness to provide the necessary support is unreliable. Students also face difficulty in recording lectures as lecturers may have a fear of being misquoted (and there are no guidelines around recording lectures). Instead, students are left to covertly capture course material without their lecturer knowing. As an interview with one student reported:

> There were some professors who didn't allow us to record the lectures. They were not from our faculty; they were from [another] faculty. But still they didn't allow us to record lectures because they were afraid that we might take anything against them … so we always try to record on a mobile phone or MP4 without taking professor permission, because this is the only solution for us to taking notes (Attia, 2009, p. 30).

Receiving course materials in an accessible format continues to be an important challenge faced by students with disabilities. Although the 2013 Marrakesh Treaty aimed to reduce the global shortage of print materials in special accessible formats for persons who are blind, vision impaired or have other print disabilities, most universities refuse to provide a soft copy (word or PDF) in order to ensure copyright (USAID, 2017). As most of the professors sell their books to the students, they have a fear that the Egyptian copyright laws will not protect their rights in case of plagiarism.

While there are disability support units existing in some universities in Egypt, Jordan and other Middle-Eastern countries, they use different methods to support their students. As a result, some universities may lack important types of support required by students with disabilities, such as Braille printing or providing them with module books with accessible formats to suit their impairments. What makes this even more difficult is when funding resources allocated to provide this support is minimal. Due to the lack of systematic support, some students with disabilities used their own creativity to gather support, relying on their friends, disability NGOs or other sorts of accommodation. This extra effort should not be their responsibility, but rather that of the higher education institution.

Universities must establish support service offices so that students are not left to their own devices. This is a form of discrimination. Applying some consistent monitoring and evaluation mechanisms from the Ministry of Higher Education may guarantee efficient and equitable support.

All universities should be required to deliver their course materials and/or reading lists in an appropriate accessible format. In addition, clear permission should be given to students with disabilities to record the lectures after taking consent that this will be only for their own use. Protecting the rights of university staff's published books and articles must be balanced with the students' needs for equal access.

EXAM TIME ARRANGEMENTS

Exams are particularly stressful for most university students (Nagpal et al., 2015; Sansgiry & Sail, 2006). They are even more difficult for students with disabilities as there is invariably inadequate access to the necessary accommodations to meet their needs. University regulations lack clarity with regards to exam time extension; providing personal assistance with a necessary capacity to type for students with disabilities; providing the exam questions in an appropriate format; and so on. As a result, Egyptian universities follow different arbitrary methods when organizing their exam arrangements (Attia, 2009). For example, some universities use oral exams for vision impaired students while others give the students the opportunity to use a computer to sit their exams independently. Yet other universities provide a personal assistant to write for the students. This un-systematic approach creates inequality in the evaluation process among students with disabilities studying the same courses in different universities.

During my undergraduate study, I required someone to dictate during my exam. Practice in that specific institution was to write a request to the department each term asking them to assign a personal assistant. It was up to them whether I received this accommodation or not.

Sometimes the assigned person was not necessarily capable to read and write for us. Senior management had a ready answer to any complaint by me, or a fellow student: "we have to provide you with someone who is in lower education than your degree so he cannot answer the question for you." On one occasion, at the beginning of a French exam, the personal assistant assigned to me confessed: "to be honest with you, I cannot read or write French". This, of course, begs the question about the basic qualifications of the personal assistants who write for students with disabilities, as well as the value placed on the service (and students) by senior management.

Clear and structured exam arrangements are required. Consulting with students with disabilities who are aware of their needs will inform the university as to the best way to respond to them without violating the integrity of assessment. Simple practices such as designing the exam to suit everyone including students with disabilities will also be useful to improve this structure. It is important for higher education institutions to provide reasonable accommodation such as time, qualified PAs and computer software if necessary to ensure exam equality. All exam accommodation and arrangement should be done by the university. This will largely reduce the stress that disabled students have when handling this themselves each semester.

CONCLUSION

The issue of including students with disabilities in higher education in the majority world goes beyond merely having some ramps and accessible toilets. It is about re-examining and restructuring university cultures, ensuring that all university students can access what they require to have equal academic and social wellbeing during their studies. The ad hoc nature of admissions and supports must change. Policies about higher education must be developed to support the majority world context. These should then be communicated with university staff, with guidance and training on putting these into practice. Each university must have a clear equality and diversity policy ensuring that all its members can access university life. Structuring a stronger co-operation between the ministry of higher education and the civil community working in the field of disability can provide some hands-on expertise to better benefit the students with disabilities.

For disabled students to overcome the existing multitude of barriers, they may rely on various alternatives to structure their own reasonable accommodations. They could rely on friends, volunteers or external support. Using their networks and being flexible and charismatic may assist them to pursue this aim. The existing solidarity within Egyptian communities could also facilitate receiving support from their families. Some studies reported a high level of achievement of students with disabilities, despite the inaccessibility of the higher education environment—a case that is even more prevalent in the majority world (Groce, 2018). It is hoped that this can this can provide some guidance and encouragement to any student with disability in higher education.

Policies and decrees that govern students with disabilities in higher education not only differ from country to country, but also nationally between different universities. Egyptian national disability policies missed essential support schemes when they were developed, such as personal assistance and note taking and which exist in many minority world universities. This has negatively affected students with disabilities' university life. The 2003 Egyptian accessibility building code may require further attention and monitoring. Currently, inaccessible environments stand as a barrier to students with physical disabilities accessing departments.

This section analysis suggests that multiple factors are required to achieve the inclusivity of higher education. Not only careful consideration and innovative solutions from institutions, but also university cultures that stress inclusion at both the macro and micro levels, along with a political space that allows disabled people to express their voices and demands.

REFERENCES

Attia, M. (2009). *Barriers facing students with disabilities in Egyptian universities: The experience of visually impaired students* (Unpublished master's thesis). University of Leeds, Leeds, UK.

Constitute Project. (2014). *Egypt's constitution of 2014*. Retrieved from https://www.constituteproject.org/constitution/Egypt_2014

Education, Audiovisual and Culture Executive Agency (EACEA). (2018). *Egypt country profile*. Retrieved from http://eacea.ec.europa.eu/tempus/participating_countries/impact/egypt.pdf

Goode, J. (2007). "Managing" disability: Early experiences of university students with disabilities. *Disability and Society*, 22(1), 35–48.

Groce, N. E. (2018, July 1). Global disability: An emerging issue. *Global Health*. Retrieved from https://www.thelancet.com/journals/langlo/article/PIIS2214-109X(18)30265-1/fulltext

International Disability Alliance (IDA). (2016). *The 2030 Agenda: The inclusion of persons with disabilities: Comprehensive guide*. Retrieved from https://www.internationaldisabilityalliance.org/sites/default/files/documents/2030_agenda_comprehensive_guide_for_persons_with_disabilities_comp.pdf

Law on the Rights of Persons with Disabilities. Law No. 10 of 2018 (EG).

Matshedisho, K. J. (2007). Access to higher education for students with disabilities in South Africa: A contradictory conjuncture of benevolence, rights and the social model of disability. *Disability & Society*, 22(7), 685–699.

Ministry of Higher Education, Egypt. (1972). *Law no. 49 on the organisation of universities*. Retrieved from https://bu.edu.eg/BUNews/136

Mittermaier, A. (2014). "Bread, Freedom, Social Justice: The Egyptian Uprising and a Sufi Khidma." *Cultural Anthropology*, 29(1), 54–79.

Nagpal, S., Grewal, S., Walia, L., & Kaur, V. (2015). A study to access the exam stress in medical college and various stressors contributing to exam stress. *Scholars Journal of Applied Medical Sciences (SJAMS)*, 3(7c), 2615–2620.

National Tempus Office (TEMPUS), undated. *Egypt country profile*. Retrieved from http://eacea.ec.europa.eu/tempus/participating_countries/impact/egypt.pdf

Nagata, K. K. (2007). Disability and development: Is the rights model of disability valid in the Arab region? An evidence-based field survey in Lebanon and Jordan. *Asia Pacific Disability Rehabilitation Journal*, 19(1), 60–78.

New Law for Persons with Disabilities. [Online]. Retrieved from http://en.wataninet.com/politics/new-law-for-persons-with-disability/23162/. Accessed 28 June 2018.

Salmi, J., & Bassett, R. M. (2012). Opportunities for all? The equity challenge in tertiary education. *World Bank*. Retrieved from https://www.salzburgglobal.org/fileadmin/user_upload/Documents/2010-2019/2012/495/Session_Document_OpportunitiesforAll_495.pdf

Sansgiry, S. S., & Sail, K. (2006). Effect of students' perceptions of course load on test anxiety. *American Journal of Pharmaceutical Education*, 70(2), 26. Retrieved from https://www.ncbi.nlm.nih.gov/pmc/articles/PMC1636912/

USAID. (2017). *Needs assessment of persons with disabilities in Egyptian public universities and regional technical colleges: Final report*. Retrieved from https://dec.usaid.gov/dec/content/Detail_Presto.aspx?ctID=ODVhZjk4NWQtM2YyMi00YjRmLTkxNjktZTcxMjM2NDBmY2Uy&rID=MjM2OTYw

CHAPTER 12

A Hierarchy of Impairments: The Absence of Body Size in Disability Accommodations Within Universities

ERIN PRITCHARD

Access is something some people have and some don't. (Titchkosky, 2008, p. 3)

INTRODUCTION

Over the past 30 years, there has been an increase in the provision of disability accommodations within the built environment. This is due to the shift in the understanding of disability from a medical perspective to a social constructivist one. A medical-model understanding perceives disability to be the deficit of the disabled person; in order to fit in with the rest of society, they must be "fixed." The social model, on the other hand, argues that disability is the result of a society that does not take into account the needs of people with impairments (Oliver, 1990). According to the Union of Impaired People Against Segregation (UPIAS), disability is something imposed on people with impairments: "Disability is the disadvantage or restriction of activity caused by contemporary social organisation, which takes little or no account of people who have physical impairments," (UPIAS, 1976, p. 14)—although it must be acknowledged that impairments are not only physical, but can also include sensory, learning and mental impairments.

This shift in how disability is understood has led to the need to change built environments. The disability rights movement can be credited with many of the changes in the treatment towards disabled people, including the provision of disabled facilities and spaces (Bickenbach et al., 1999). Policies and legislation, such as the Americans with Disabilities Act (1990) and section 504 of the Rehabilitation Act of 1973 (1978) in the US, and the Disability Discrimination Act (1995) and Equality Act (2010) in the UK, which were a response to disability activism, have aided in responding to some access needs of disabled people, and thus provided more disabled people with the opportunity to access higher education. However, access provisions have not responded to the diverse range of disabled people entering higher education.

Specifically, these provisions have failed to address how higher-education administrators sometimes perceive disability. If a student is not perceived to be sufficiently disabled, they will not be provided with the accommodations they request. This is partly due to policies and legislation only requiring minimum standards to be met and due to perceptions of what disability can be. It is the notion of *who* is disabled that affects the implementation of suitable spaces and facilities for a range of disabled people (Cooper, 1997). Body sizes that exceed the norm are often not considered to be disabled, despite the fact that the built environment is created for the average-sized person. The materiality of spaces can be disabling for people whose body size does not adhere to average standards (Longhurst, 2010).

My impairment is dwarfism. The built environment that is created for the average-sized person creates many disabling barriers for me. Everyday facilities, such as door handles, are literally out of reach. Dwarfism is categorised in a person "who is no taller than 4ft 10" (147cm). I am 4ft (122cm), the average stature for someone with dwarfism. My precise impairment is Achondroplasia, the most common form of dwarfism. This form of dwarfism results in a disproportionate body size; my torso is of average stature, while my limbs are much smaller. Terms used to refer to a person with dwarfism often differ from person to person and within different countries. I have chosen here to use the term "person with dwarfism" as it aids in demonstrating how the built environment is not size-appropriate, i.e., I am "dwarfed" by spaces and facilities made for the average-sized person, which is disabling. However, dwarfism, as well as other body sizes that break from the norm, is contested as a disability, resulting in the lack of suitable accommodations. To be provided with accommodations, I have often had to prove my disability and demonstrate why certain accommodations are important for me.

This chapter argues that body size as a disability has been largely ignored, resulting in the creation of a hierarchy of impairments in providing disability access within universities. This chapter demonstrates how physical disability access largely revolves around wheelchair users, ignoring the needs of people with body sizes that are outside the norm. Within the standard university lecture theatre, for example, there is now a removable set of seats to accommodate wheelchair users, but there is no seating that is actually size-suitable for a range of body sizes. This chapter calls for more inclusion of body size when providing disability accommodations within universities. It highlights what universities should provide for students with a body size that differs to the norm.

THE QUEST FOR ACCESS

Adjusting to university life can be difficult for all students. For disabled students, this is often made more challenging due to having to manage accommodations (Getzel & Thoma, 2008), while there is no guarantee that that those accommodations will be suitable or even provided. Disabled students can be discouraged from pursuing a degree due to the problems associated with access that they are likely to encounter (Hannam-Swan, 2018).

In order to receive appropriate support, disabled people must first prove the extent of their perceived limitation and in need of accommodations (Olney & Brockelman, 2003). This can be difficult when an impairment is contested as a disability. Attitudes towards different impairments vary within society, creating a *hierarchy* (Deal, 2003). This includes what people consider an impairment to be, which results in some impairments being more widely accommodated for than others. As a result, a student whose body size differs from the norm is disabled by a society that builds for this convention.

Every country has its own procedure for providing disability accommodations. In the USA, universities should adhere to the Americans with Disabilities Act (Ada.gov., 2018) by providing reasonable accommodations if the student is able to prove their disability. In the UK and Canada, grants are also available for students who are able to prove that they have a disability. Students in the UK are often provided with funds to cover the costs associated with their disability through Disabled Students Allowance (DSA). DSA has been criticised for taking an individualised perception of disability, which goes against a wider social understanding of disability (Riddell et al., 2005). While these funds may provide the economic means to buy assistive devices or to pay for personal help recommended by disability support, they do not cover the costs of providing the right facilities, including accessible infrastructure. Providing accommodating infrastructure would reduce the need for costly assistive devices, which are not always suitable. It may often feel like the accommodations that are provided are more suitable for another impairment. For example, I was provided with a Dictaphone, technology usually used by students with dyslexia, to record lectures as the lecture seating was unsuitable for my size and made writing difficult. Provisions like these act like a pacifier and resist changing what is really disabling—in this case, the university seating -- as the adjustments required are deemed unnecessary or too costly. In the United States, it is the responsibility of the student to advocate for accommodations. Staff and faculty members will then liaise and decide on accommodations for the student. This can be problematic, as the staff and faculty members may not have the right knowledge concerning the disabled student's needs.

When starting university, there is no guarantee that all accommodations will be put in place. While discussing accommodations, students should ask for a time frame of when they will be completed, in the form a written report. Not being provided with appropriate accommodations when starting a degree can impede one's ability to fully participate. Disabled students have reported being "time-disadvantaged" through obstacles presented in arranging accommodations and getting them implemented (Seymour & Hunter, 1998). Having to spend extra time trying to deal with inaccessible spaces, and constantly having to contact disability support over what should be considered minor access issues, can lead to being time-disadvantaged. Making the university's infrastructure more accommodating for a wide range of disabled people, would aid in removing some of the obstacles that create time barriers.

For example, for someone with dwarfism, a keypad entrance to a building can be a significant barrier to access. Keypads are often placed at an inaccessible height, which can in the person with dwarfism spending weeks waiting and contacting disability support, asking to have the keypad lowered in order to be able to access the building independently. The majority of facilities in a university can be either lowered or height-adjustable, depending on how they are constructed.

(IN)ACCESSIBLE INFRASTRUCTURE—AN HIERARCHY OF IMPAIRMENTS

It is a common misperception that the built environment is designed and constructed in the correct way, and that disabled people merely pose a costly problem. Spaces and facilities are designed to accommodate for a particular body standard.

> There is a tendency for architects to design and construct spaces to specific technical standards and dimensions, which revolve around the conception of the "normal" body, creating physical barriers for anyone who does not fit this conception (Imrie, 1996, p. 281).

This conception of the "normal" body has resulted in the need for disabled spaces and facilities to be added to the built environment. However, these spaces often neglect the need to accommodate for body sizes that differ from the norm (Steinfeld & Maisel, 2012).

The way disability has been accommodated within higher education is through specific adjustments that provide minimal access for a narrow range of disabled people. While many people may think of disabled students as being wheelchair users (Chard & Couch, 1998), wheelchair users make up less than 10% of the disabled population. A ramp does not provide access for all, but is merely a token gesture that adheres to minimal access standards.

Buildings often only comply with minimal guidelines, such as the requirement to provide an accessible toilet, wider entrances and ramps. While this may provide a degree of access to wheelchair users, these accommodations are not always accessible for people with dwarfism, as they are either not low enough or are too wide (Pritchard, 2015). Simply lowering items with wheelchair users in mind does not solve problems with accessibility. At one university, the supposedly accessible self-service scanner in the library proved to be problematic. The Disability Support service stated that the self-service scanner complied with the Disability Discrimination Act (1995), as it is accessible for wheelchair users. In other words, the scanner complied with a limited form of legislation meant to provide access for all disabled people, one that in reality is biased towards those with mobility impairments. To push for better access, students must be more forthright and demonstrate how not providing a more accommodating solution will impact their studies. If students are unable to take out books, their work and subsequently their grades will be affected. Through demonstrating how they are at a disadvantage to other students, disabled students can show how they are being discriminated against and require alternative access.

An accessible physical environment can be achieved through audits and ensuring new infrastructure complies with disability regulations (Adams & Brown, 2006). However, what these regulations consider to be a disability can affect access for various impairments. Disability legislation in the UK, Hannam-Swan (2018) suggests, only caters to needs that are deemed acceptable. This creates a hierarchy of need by denying voice to those with impairments that are not deemed "acceptable." Requesting modes of access that are not recognised by the institutionis seen as unacceptable, as if asking for too much. Titchkosky calls this type of defence a "sensible say-able," which serves to make the university's lack of disability access ordinary and discourages challenge from the disabled person (2008, cited in Hannam-Swan, 2018, p. 140). "Sensible say-able" implies that inaccessibility, or accessibility for only a stereotypical disability, is what is acceptable and true in society. It justifies inaccessibility, instead of recognising that inaccessibility is a product of society and can be overcome through design that is more thoughtful. The lack of recognition of body size as a disability allows others to justify a lack of access through claiming that disability access has already been provided through the implementation of disabled facilities for one part of the disabled population.

ARE YOU SITTING COMFORTABLY?

Having the right seating is important to ensure that students are able to learn and engage effectively. If seating is uncomfortable or difficult to use, it can affect a student's performance. For someone whose body size is outside the norm, seating can prove to be very disabling (Hettrick & Attig, 2009; Huff, 2009). The mass production of facilities, including seating, is based on the premise that a person's body can adapt in order to fit (Huff, 2009). Someone who is fat, for example, may have to squeeze into some seating, which can be very uncomfortable, and even result in pain and embarrassment (Hettrick & Attig, 2009). (The term "fat" is used here as opposed to "obese" or "large," as it corresponds to accepted terminology within fat studies. Fat studies is an interdisciplinary subject, that does not focus on weight loss, but rather recognises that fatness is a human characteristic (Rothblum & Solovay, 2009). Fat studies challenges the oppression fat people experience in society, including the lack of access to spaces and facilities that accommodate for fat people. It falls in line with disability advocacy in campaigning for better access for a range of people.)

Just because a person is able to sit on a chair does not mean it is suitable for their body size. Correct posture involves being able to place the feet flat on the floor and being able to rest the elbows on the desk in front. Unless seating that is more suitable is provided, this is impossible for people with dwarfism. Most lecture theatres are made up of rows of identically fixed seating. Having to sit in incorrectly-sized chairs can be painful, and thus it is important to ensure students receive the correct seating for their body size. If students are unable to sit comfortably, then disability support should be notified.

CONCLUSION: ACCESSIBILITY FOR ALL

Disability access is not effective in providing suitable access for body sizes that deviate from the norm. A more diverse recognition of disability is needed in order to provide more accommodating infrastructure. This lack of diversity has led to a hierarchy of impairments, resulting in some impairments being more accommodated for than others. Universities need to include a larger range of impairments in their accommodations. Regarding infrastructure, more consideration needs to be given to those whose body size differs from the norm to provide better access for a wider range of disabled students.

All universities should ensure that the needs of people whose body size differs from the norm are taken into account. They need to consider facilities that are adjustable for a range of body sizes, or install one or two at different heights in order to accommodate for the very tall and small. The institution should not assume that just because a facility is suitable for one group of disabled people (such as wheelchair users), that it will be for all disabled people.

Universities and prospective students need to consider the various barriers that will be encountered. In terms of seating, consider the following: Is it wide enough, low enough? Will seats need a footrest and/or backrest? Can all students fit into a seat comfortably without it pinching? Can all students reach the table in front of them without it causing discomfort? Would the student benefit from a height-adjustable chair? Are tables easy to access? Do any drawing boards need to be lower? Can door handles be reached and are any keypad/ swipe card entrances reachable without difficulty? Are the doors too heavy to open? On staircases, can the stair rail be reached? This is an important safety aspect of any stairwell, especially in the event of a fire.

On elevators, can all students reach the buttons for all floors? Are there any services for disabled people, such as library support aiding in fetching books? Can the self-service scanner be reached? Are eBooks available? Can students be served easily in campus eating places or is a low-level service desk needed? Is there any accessible accommodation available? Is the wardrobe accessible? Is there a useful facility available, which provides a lever to bring down clothes from a high rail? Is the shower accessible? Are the kitchen facilities low enough to reach? Are restroom sinks accessible? Can all students get into the toilet cubicle without difficulty and reach the lock? Can they reach the hand dryers?

While prospective students can visit a campus and the various spaces, they will most likely to use, such as their department and student accommodation, universities should pre-empt any future difficulty for them by thoroughly assessing their spaces to ensure their campuses are truly accessible for any wishing to further their education.

REFERENCES

Ada.gov. (2018). *Americans with Disabilities Act of 1990, Aa amended with ADA Amendments Act of 2008*. [Online] Retrieved from http://www.ada.gov/pubs/adastatute08.htm#12102

Adams, M., & Brown, S. (2006). Introduction. In M. Adams & S. Brown (Eds.), *Towards inclusive learning in higher education* (pp. 1–9). London, UK: Routledge.

Bickenbach, J. E., Chatterji, S., Badley, E. M., & Ustun, T. B. (1999). Models of disablement, universalism and the international classification of impairments, disabilities and handicaps. *Social Science and Medicine, 48*(9), 1173–1187.

Chard, G., & Couch, R. (1998). Access to higher education for the disabled student: A building survey at the University of Liverpool. *Disability and Society, 13*(4), 603–623.

Cooper, C. (1997). Can a fat woman call herself disabled? *Disability and Society, 12*(1), 31–41.

Deal, M. (2003). Disabled people's attitudes towards other impairment groups: A hierarchy of impairments. *Disability and Society, 18*(7), 897–910.

Getzel, E. E., & Thoma, C. A. (2008). Experiences of college students with disabilities and the importance of self-determination in higher education settings. *Career Development and Transition for Exceptional Individuals, 31*(2), 77–84.

Imrie, R. (1996). *Disability and the city.* Salisbury, UK: The Baskerville Press.

Hannam-Swan, S. (2018). The additional labour of a PhD student. *Disability and Society, 33*(1), 138–142.

Hettrick, A., & Attig, D. (2009). Sitting pretty: Fat bodies, classroom desks and academic excess, In E. Rothblum, & S. Solovay (Eds.), *The fat studies reader* (pp. 197–204). New York, NY: New York Press.

Huff, L. J. (2009). Access to the sky: Airplane seats and fat bodies as contested spaces. In E. Rothblum & S. Solovay (Eds.), *The fat studies reader* (pp. 176–186). New York, NY: New York Press.

Legislation.gov.uk. (1995). *Disability Discrimination Act 1995.* [online]. Retrieved from http://www.legislation.gov.uk/ukpga/1995/50/introduction

Legislation.gov.uk. (2010). *Equality Act 2010.* [online]. Retrieved from http://www.legislation.gov.uk/ukpga/2010/15/contents

Longhurst, R. (2010). The disabling affects of fat: The emotional and material geographies of some women who live in Hamilton, New Zealand. In V. Chouinard, E. Hall, & R. Wilton (Eds.), *Towards enabling geographies* (pp. 199–216). Abingdon, UK: Ashgate.

Olney, M. F., & Brockelman, K. F. (2003). Out of the disability closet: Strategic use of perception management by select university students with disabilities. *Disability and Society, 18*(1), 35–50.

Oliver, M. (1990). *The politics of disablement.* London, UK: Palgrave.

Pritchard, E. (2015). The spatial experiences of dwarfs within public spaces. *Scandinavian Journal of Disability Research, 18*(3), 191–199.

Riddell, S., Tinklin, T., & Wilson, A. (2005). *Disabled students in higher education.* Abingdon, UK: Routledge.

Rothblum, E., & Solovay, S. (Eds.). (2009). *The fat studies reader.* New York, NY: New York Press.

Seymour, E., & Hunter, A. (1998). *Talking about disability: The education and work experience of graduates and undergraduates with disabilities in science, mathematics and engineering majors.* Boulder, CO: University of Colorado.

Steinfeld, E., & Maisel, L. J. (2012). *Universal design.* Hoboken, NJ: Wiley.

Titchkosky, T. (2008). "To pee or not to pee?" Ordinary talk about extraordinary exclusions in a university environment. *The Canadian Journal of Sociology, 33*(1), 37–60.

UPIAS. (1976). *Fundamental principles of disability.* London, UK: Union of Physically Impaired Against Segregation.

CHAPTER 13

"I Can't Even Reach the Waffle-Maker!": Increasing Access for Students with Physical Disabilities on University Campuses

APRIL B. COUGHLIN

INTRODUCTION

During my first year as an undergraduate student living on campus and away from home for the first time, I rolled into the residence dining hall one day and up to the counter to make a waffle. What I found was a waffle-maker out of reach—perched on top of a five-foot high counter, with no possibility of me using it independently. I rolled back to my dorm room waffle-less. The next day I went back to the cafeteria and faced the inaccessible waffle-maker again. This time, instead of feeling defeated, I felt frustrated and discriminated against. Here I was, a brand new freshman just like everyone else, but I was unable to exercise my independence and right to make my own waffles. I spoke to the manager in the dining hall who told me that the waffle-maker could not be lowered.

This fight was not over. I took the issue all the way up the chain of command to the administration. By the end of the semester, the waffle-maker had been lowered, and I had become an activist. It was a small, but important victory in the fight for equity. The university's initial denial of providing access to the waffle-maker ignited a disability advocacy fire within me, which eventually led to the fight for access to other places on campus.

This chapter considers accessibility through a disability studies lens, which puts the stories and experiences of those living with disabilities at the forefront and seeks to create a more equal, informed, and inclusive society (Baglieri & Shapiro,

2012; Linton, 1998). Disability studies aims to eliminate barriers (architectural, policies, procedures and attitudes) that disable people, rather than positioning the disability solely as an impairment within the individual or a problem in need of fixing (Baglieri & Shapiro, 2012). From living on campus, to accessing classrooms and extracurricular activities in higher education, examples of environmental and social barriers paint the backdrop of the segregation that many students with physical impairments face. In response to these barriers, many students begin to identify more strongly with their impairments and question university environments, policies, and procedures that work to shape their experiences. As a result, students resort to various forms of advocacy in an effort to effect change on campus and in society. This chapter acts as a guide to stimulate assertive action and to indicate instances in which students may need to fight for their right to access. It also indicates to institutions where they can preempt possible future difficulties for students with disabilities to make universities more responsive to the needs of *all* students. Specific areas discussed include choosing a university, registering as "disabled," touring campus, living in the residence halls, attending classes, and responding to inaccessibility and exclusion through advocacy.

CHOOSING A UNIVERSITY AND REGISTERING AS "DISABLED"

Type "physical accessibility" or "disabled/disability access" into any university website search engine and you will immediately be directed to the Disability Resource Center. Go a step further and it will prompt you to register with the Disability Resource Center or Office of Disability Services in order to receive accommodations. Some students see this as a welcome sign of accessibility and inclusion. Others, who do not necessarily identify strongly with their disability, view attending the university as their first chance to "start fresh" without having to be labeled in order to receive services (Brune & Wilson, 2013; Taub et al., 2004).

When wishing to live on campus, most students have to apply for housing by filling out some brief paperwork before being assigned a room in a residence hall. For students with disabilities, the process can be much more complicated, often requiring paperwork signed by a doctor with proof of medical necessity for an accessible residence. If an able-bodied student wants to have a car on campus, they merely have to go to parking services, fill out a form and pick up their permit. They do not have to get examined by a doctor in order to have their application form signed.

Students with disabilities often are required to get medically examined and diagnosed in order to receive disability-related services. The systems set in place in our society require proof of disability and this "proof" almost always reverts back to a diagnosis, locating disability firmly within the medical profession (Longmore & Umansky, 2001). The medicalizing of disability through these gatekeeping practices in higher education works to further marginalize and oppress students with disabilities, which can lead to the desire to distance oneself from a disability identity altogether (Sauer & Kasa, 2012). It is also incredibly time consuming and expensive for students to continually see a doctor in order to get these forms (among many others) signed.

Students must not be afraid to speak up and question these pathologizing practices related to non-medical aspects of university life and even inquire if there are alternatives to being seen by a doctor to complete the paperwork. While it is important for institutions to have checks and balances, these procedures need to be made less cumbersome to disabled students. If an application for a disabled parking permit requires a doctor's signature, the university may consider reimbursing students for the appointment needed to obtain this signature or even provide on-campus medical personnel (paid for by the university) to sign off on these required forms.

UNIVERSITY COMMITMENT TO DIVERSITY AND INCLUSION

Universities often tout their commitment to diversity and inclusion in their mission statements (Meacham & Barrett, 2003; Wilson et al., 2012), but in many instances they end up leaving disability out of the equation altogether. It is crucial to question the university's commitment to access and inclusion if disability seems absent from their website. When applying to a university, students can speak with a representative to inquire about the accessibility of specific areas on campus and the university's overall commitment to inclusion and representation of students with disabilities. When institutions are designing their website, specific focus must be placed on evaluating the content for disability representation and who is included and left out, both in images and content. Campus maps on the university website must include accurate and up-to-date information about accessibility (i.e., dorms, entrances, parking, bathrooms, classrooms, study areas, eateries, and social spaces).

EXPLORING, LIVING, AND GOING TO CLASS ON CAMPUS: SEPARATE IS STILL NOT EQUAL

For many students, their first introduction to campus is through a college tour. Due to access barriers, students with physical disabilities are often led on a completely separate "accessible" tour than their non-disabled peers. Separate tours are *not* acceptable. If students find themselves in this situation on a university tour, they can demand that *all* students take the "accessible" route together.

DORMS, DINING HALLS, LAUNDRY, GARBAGE REMOVAL AND ATHLETIC FACILITIES

Whereas some universities require all first year students to live on campus, many often do not provide wheelchair accessible housing, resulting in limited choices and segregation. As a freshman living on campus, I was provided a "medical single" dorm room, which required medical proof through an examination and letter from my physician, placing disability solely within the medical model (Baglieri, 2017; Biklen, 1988). There were four residence hall complexes on campus, only one of which provided wheelchair accessible housing, where I resided. All of my non-disabled freshmen peers lived in a completely separate area of campus where they dined, studied, and socialized together. If I wanted to participate in any of these activities with my new peers, I would have to travel a half mile across campus to their residence hall.

When students with and without disabilities are not provided the opportunity to engage with one another socially, barriers are presented to relationship building (Egilson & Traustadottir, 2009; Nichols & Quaye, 2009). Universities need to consider the importance of social interactions between students in residence halls and provide accessible housing in *all* residence halls and dining facilities to ensure *all* students have equal access and enjoy the social benefits of living on campus.

At most universities, students are required to pay an activity fee, which partially funds staff and maintenance of athletic facilities. These could include gym equipment and a pool. However, many universities may not have wheelchair accessible weightlifting and exercise equipment in the gym or a chair lift into the pool. Students with disabilities should not be required to pay the full student activity fee if these services are not fully accessible to them.

While universities offer accessible dorm rooms, facilities such as vending machines, laundry rooms, and garbage removal may not be fully accessible to students with disabilities. Due to structural barriers such as stairs, heavy doors, or machines that are out of reach, students with physical disabilities may not have full independent access to such services. Instead of making these facilities fully accessible, some universities address the issue by hiring assistants to do these tasks *for* students with disabilities. As a result, individuals with disabilities are automatically placed in a marginalized position where they are forced to depend on others (Priestley, 1999). While assistants for ADLs (activities of daily living) can prove to be beneficial to many students with disabilities, this should be offered as an option in addition to an already accessible living environment. Paid assistance should not be used by the university as a band-aid for structural inaccessibility.

When registering for housing, students should inquire about the following areas: number of residence halls that are accessible and where they are located; accessible features in dorm rooms (i.e., window locks, door handles, lowered closet space); location of accessible bathrooms and showers along with a description of each (i.e., grab bars, tilted mirrors, raised toilet seats, hand-held shower heads, shower chairs); dining hall access (i.e., lowered counters, tables, self-serve areas); laundry facilities (i.e., top or front loading washers and dryers); vending machines with lowered buttons and payment slot; garbage removal location (i.e., weight of door to garbage removal room and height of garbage shoot).

ATTENDING CLASS

As a college freshman, I entered the lecture hall only to see five hundred seats with steps leading down to the front on both sides. There was no sign of a ramp. The "accessible" seating was located all the way in the back of the room with very few spots for a wheeler to fit. I thought to myself, "What if I need to speak to the professor or do a class presentation? How would I get down there?" I immediately began advocating for increased building accessibility on campus.

Physical barriers on campus can limit access to academic opportunities. These include heavy doors that prevent students from physically getting through and entering buildings, as well as inaccessible lecture halls and classroom spaces. Lecture halls that are not ramped force students with mobility disabilities to sit all the way in the back or directly in the front of the room. Lack of access limits students' seating choice, and physically separates students with disabilities from their non-disabled peers and instructors, preventing them from engaging fully in class activities. There is no reason why a learning space cannot be made fully accessible to *all* users. Institutions of higher education spend thousands of dollars each year on updated technology and user-friendly furniture for these spaces, but often there is little to no consideration for whether the spaces themselves are physically accessible to *all* users to begin with.

OTHER ISSUES OF ACCESS ON CAMPUS: BATHROOMS, SIGNAGE, PARKING AND GRADUATION

As a graduate student learning about inclusive education, I routinely left class to use the bathroom. My journey usually took a half hour in total and began by putting my jacket on. I pushed my chair down the long hallway of the third floor from one end of the building to the other, took the elevator down to the first floor and pushed to the other end of the building to the main exit. I rolled out into the snow, ice, or rain, pushed down the sidewalk, across the street, up the curb cut, and into a coffee shop. This was where the closest wheelchair accessible bathroom was located near campus. I then started my journey back to class, having missed a half hour of valuable instruction.

In this section I offer various methods for responding to issues of inaccessibility on campus. These include creating fully accessible bathrooms, improving signage and information about accessibility, updating language on existing signage, providing and enforcing accessible parking, and ensuring access for all at commencement ceremonies. Every person should have the right to use the bathroom in the university building they are in. No one should be required to exit the building, roll down the street, and go into another business just to exercise that right. Inaccessible bathrooms are not only inconvenient, but they also send the message to students with physical disabilities that "Your needs are not equal to those who do not require an accessible bathroom stall." If bathrooms on campus are not accessible, universities must make an immediate plan and commitment to address this. Students with disabilities must raise the issue with administration if their right to bathroom access is denied.

Signage goes a long way in the search for access and time spent looking for entrances, bathrooms, and elevators on campus. However, posting a sign that says "accessible" does not automatically make something accessible. Signage needs to be accurate. If students notice signage for access is missing or needs to be replaced, they can contact the administration with a photo and description of the location along with a written request for improvements. Students need to follow up on their requests and always keep a printed or digital copy of all communications as a reference. Institutions must allocate funds for improving accessibility, which includes increased and updated signage. Signage is an easy (and inexpensive) thing to get *right*.

Accessible parking is essential for individuals with disabilities. These spaces need to be kept clear of garbage bins, snow piles, and university issued vehicles. Some campuses are updating language on signage for these parking spaces from "handicapped parking" to "parking for persons with disabilities" or placing the accessible icon logo on a sign that says "reserved." By changing the words or symbols on entrances, bathrooms, and parking signage, we can work to change the way disability is perceived in society (DePoy & Gilson, 2010; Wilson & Lewiecki-Wilson, 2003). This is also a great way to take the lead in creating a progressive, positive, and welcoming disability culture on campus.

Many graduation ceremonies are inaccessible to students with physical disabilities because of no ramps. By providing only steps at graduations, universities continually privilege the able-bodied majority over individuals with physical impairments. This is ableism in action. Rauscher and McClintock (1996) define ableism as "a pervasive system of discrimination and exclusion that oppresses people who have mental, emotional and physical disabilities (p. 198)." Ableist decisions at the university create an "alienating and oppressive built environment" (Imrie, 1998, p. 131) which serve as hostile acts of exclusion that force students to be isolated and unseen (von Tippelskirch & Linton, 2014) from their non-disabled peers. The burden is automatically placed on students to check with the university ahead of time to ensure commencement will be accessible. Non-disabled students do not have to check prior to graduation to make sure that the stage will be accessible for them to cross. By including ramps at every graduation ceremony, physical access for everyone is guaranteed.

ADVOCATING FOR CHANGE

University is where students with disabilities can develop into disability rights advocates (Barnes, 2007). Away from home and facing constant obstacles to inclusion, students often begin to recognize injustices such as those I have discussed in this chapter, and work to resist them. When buildings and classrooms are inaccessible to those with physical disabilities, universities turn to familiar justifications like lack of funding in the budget for renovations. This is what Titchkosky (2008) calls "justifiable exclusion" (p. 46) which works to further marginalize and discount individuals with disabilities in our society. One advocacy method is letter writing. While effective, letters often get piled up on administrators' desks or buried in their email inbox and forgotten about or dismissed because of more pressing matters. Phone calls are an effective strategy, but are often sent to voicemail where messages may not be heard. Video activism is another tool for gaining the attention of university administration and effecting change. Video creates the opportunity to provide information from the user's point of view and can convey the message in a more accessible and immediate way than a letter or memo. Videos can also reach a wider viewing audience when posted on the Internet and as a result, bring these issues to the forefront.

Institutions must utilize the expertise of individuals with disabilities when making decisions about access on campus. Before building or remodeling, it is essential to gather input from the users themselves through creating a task force consisting of students, faculty, and staff with disabilities that specifically advises the university on accessibility issues. At the same time, students do not have to wait for universities to invite them to serve on task forces in order to have an impact. Student-led coalitions can be very effective in advocating for change on campus. Student voice matters.

CONCLUDING THOUGHTS

When I began as an undergraduate, I never could have imagined how my experiences with inaccessibility and marginalization would shape the disability advocate and activist that I have become today. At the time, I was just trying to socialize with my new peers, access my classes, do my own laundry, and independently make a waffle in the dining hall. I now view these barriers to full participation at the university as violations of my rights as a person with a disability. As a fully enrolled student, I was not receiving the same access to services as my ablebodied peers. While there are many battles to fight and the work for equity gets tiring, it is not sufficient to just passively accept these injustices, nor is it enough to just solve your own situation and be content with that. Students with disabilities must actively demand access and permanent changes to be implemented in the ways universities provide access and services to *all* students. Ableist practices are in every facet of life and this is evidenced by the pervasive physical inaccessibility that exists in educational institutions (Connor & Coughlin, 2016; Danforth, 2014; Siebers, 2008). Ironically, these are the very spaces where the greatest examples of access, forward thinking, and inclusive practices should be exhibited. Students with disabilities need to be actively involved in resisting inequity and advocating for the right to full access and experience at universities. Institutions need to recognize the injustices that exist in regard to access and respond to these by taking immediate steps to address barriers to full participation, while utilizing the input of students and faculty with disabilities on campus. In order to create truly inclusive university campuses, we need to go beyond lip service about the need for increasing access. Universities must commit the resources and the will to make equitable access a reality for *all* students.

REFERENCES

Baglieri, S. (2017). *Disability studies and the inclusive classroom: Critical practices for embracing diversity in education*. New York, NY: Routledge.

Baglieri, S., & Shapiro, A. (2012). *Disability studies and the inclusive classroom: Critical practices for creating least restrictive attitudes*. New York, NY: Routledge.

Barnes, C. (2007). Disability, higher education and the inclusive society. *British Journal of Sociology of Education, 28*(1), 135–145.

Biklen, D. (1988). The myth of clinical judgment. *Journal of Social Issues, 44*(1), 127–140.

Brune, J. A., & Wilson, D. J. (2013). *Disability and passing: Blurring the lines of identity*. Philadelphia, PA: Temple University Press.

Connor, D. J., & Coughlin, A. B. (2016). Ramping it up: Calling attention to dis/ability at the end of education's social contract. In R. Malhotra (Ed.), *Disability politics in a global economy: Essays in honor of Marta Russell* (pp. 118–134). New York, NY: Routledge.

Danforth, S. (Ed.). (2014). *Becoming a great inclusive educator*. New York, NY: Peter Lang.
DePoy, E., & Gilson, G. (2010). Disability design and branding: Rethinking disability within the 21st Century. *Disability Studies Quarterly*, *30*(2). Retrieved from http://dsq-sds.org/article/view/1247/1274
Egilson, S. T., & Traustadottir, R. (2009). Participation of students with physical disabilities in the school environment. *The American Journal of Occupational Therapy*, *63*(3), 264–272.
Imrie, R. (1998). Oppression, disability and access in the built environment. In T. Shakespeare (Ed.), *The disability reader* (pp. 129–146). New York, NY: Continuum.
Linton, S. (1998). *Claiming disability: Knowledge and identity*. New York, NY: New York University Press.
Longmore, P. K., & Umansky, L. (2001). *The new disability history: American perspectives*. New York, NY: New York University Press.
Meacham, J., & Barrett, C. (2003). Commitment to diversity in institutional mission statements. *Diversity Digest*, *7*(1–2), 6–9.
Nichols, A. H., & Quaye, S. J. (2009). Beyond accommodation: Removing barriers to academic and social engagement for students with disabilities. In S. J. Quaye & S. R. Harper (Eds.), *Student engagement in higher education: Theoretical perspectives and practical approaches for diverse populations* (pp. 39–60). New York, NY: Routledge.
Priestley, M. (1999). Discourse and identity: Disabled children in mainstream high schools. In M. Corker & S. French (Eds.), *Disability discourse* (pp. 92–102). Buckingham, UK: Open University Press.
Rauscher, L., & McClintock, J. (1996). Ableism curriculum design. In M. Adams, L. A. Bell, & P. Griffen (Eds.), *Teaching for diversity and social justice* (pp. 198–231). New York, NY: Routledge.
Sauer, J. S., & Kasa, C. (2012). Preservice teachers listen to families of students with disabilities and learn a disability studies stance. *Issues in Teacher Education*, *21*(2), 165–183.
Siebers, T. (2008). *Disability theory*. Ann Arbor, MI: University of Michigan Press.
Taub, D. E., McLorg, P. A., & Fanflik, P. L. (2004). Stigma management strategies among women with physical disabilities: Contrasting approaches of downplaying or claiming a disability status. *Deviant Behavior*, *25*(2), 169–190.
Titchkosky, T. (2008). "To Pee or Not to Pee?": Ordinary talk about extraordinary exclusions in a university environment. *Canadian Journal of Sociology*, *33*(1), 37–60.
von Tippelskirch, C. (Producer & Director), & Linton, S. (Producer). (2014). *Invitation to dance* [Motion picture]. USA: Metuffer Films.
Wilson, J. C., & Lewiecki-Wilson, C. (2003). *Embodied rhetorics: Disability in language and culture*. Carbondale, IL: Southern Illinois University Press.
Wilson, J. L., Meyer, K. A., & McNeal, L. (2012). Mission and diversity statements: What they do and do not say. *Innovative Higher Education*, *37*(2), 125–139.

CHAPTER 14

Assistance Dogs and Academia: Supporting the Dynamic Duo in the post-COVID "New World"

DR. G. GELLER AND DR. A. MÜLLER

INTRODUCTION

This chapter is about the inclusiveness of Assistance Dogs on campus. It focuses on anti-discrimination legislation the Disability Discrimination Act (Commonwealth) (Commonwealth of Australia, 1992),varying Equal Opportunity Acts in Australia (e.g., Government of NSW, 1977; Government of South Australia, 1984; Victorian Equal Opportunity & Equal Rights Commission, 2017) and supporting the physical and mental health needs of students. Stressors for students with assistance dogs include being a source of public attention, being approached to pat the working dog, refusal of entry, and navigating the public space while meeting the needs of two entities (Gravrok et al., 2019; Tsang et al., 2021). These issues require immediate attention by universities—now even more so in the aftermath of the COVID-19 pandemic. The pandemic has contributed to greater anxieties within the Assistance Dog Handler communities, and this ranges from difficulties with class attendance to potential hand sanitiser toxicity to Assistance Dogs. Wearing masks is also an area that needs to be considered, because this impacts the communication between Assistance Dog and Handler and also requires the Assistance Dog to be desensitised to the space. Finally, isolation also affects the training level of the dog.

First and foremost, this chapter maintains that universities do not always meet the needs of students with Assistance Dogs (Guide, Hearing and Service

Dogs), and we call for change. Although situated in Australia, we think universities elsewhere should pay attention to our experiences. We consider the legislative space that we live in and examine the inclusiveness of Assistance Dogs on campus. We explore concepts such as discrimination and how to support the physical and mental health needs of students, and we highlight areas that require sustained consideration. We also examine the teaching perspective and how this evolved pre- and post-pandemic. We consider positive experiences associated with online learning, and the nexus between this and Assistance Dogs. We argue that meeting university deadlines during lockdowns without consideration of our Assistance Dogs has had far reaching consequences in terms of productivity, and impacted on students not being able to meet their own needs. We consider this and other tensions that surround the workspace and then move on to how an Assistance Dog in the online teaching environment can be beneficial for both Handlers as students. Finally, we explore the mental anguish that discrimination can have to a student who utilizes an Assistance Dog in their medical treatment, and the long-term consequences this can have from their experiences at the university if faced with direct or indirect discrimination. We position ourselves within this chapter as dis-abled Masters and PhD students, university lecturers, canine behaviourists that specialize in Assistance Dog training and accreditation, and as healthcare professionals.

YOUR SPACE IS ALSO OUR SPACE

An Assistance Dog is considered to be a disability aid—one that is specifically trained to provide support to people that have a disabling condition (Tsang et al., 2021). These conditions can include hearing or vision impairments, mental illness, seizures, and autism. There are generally three categories that Assistance Dogs can be grouped into: Guide Dogs, Hearing Dogs, and Service Dogs. Service Dogs can be further categorised into the following: Mobility Assistance Dogs, Seizure Alert Dogs, Medic Alert Dogs, and Psychiatric Service Dogs (Geller, 2018). Assistance Dogs in Australia have very specific "rights", namely the right of public access (Geller, 2018). This means that trained Assistance Dogs are allowed in public places and on public passenger vehicles (Commonwealth of Australia, 1992; Human Rights Commission, 2016). Businesses such as restaurants, hotels, shops, taxis, theatres, and sports facilities must not refuse entry to Assistance Dogs, and strict penalties apply if access is refused. This holds true in other jurisdictions such as the United States of America and the United Kingdom (Commonwealth of Australia, 1992; Human Rights Commission, 2016; UK Government, 2010; US Department of Justice, 2010).

In Australia, the Human Rights Commission (2016) oversees discriminatory matters, which includes the discrimination Assistance Dogs and their handlers may encounter while in public. Elsewhere, the Equality and Human Rights Commission (2018) oversees these matters in Great Britain, while in the United States the Civil Rights Division of the Department of Justice (2017) does so. In Australia, the Human Rights Commission (2016) is charged with taking complaints and mediating on behalf of consumers. Should mediation fail, then the Federal Court is engaged. Whilst there remain a dearth of scholarly studies that explore discrimination surrounding Assistance Dogs, the Human Rights Commission (2016) have been collating the number of complaints related to Assistance Dogs. The Commission has received an increasing number of complaints, specifically to do with Assistance Dogs other than Guide Dogs.

Direct discrimination means that a person is treated less favourable because of their "protected characteristics", disability is one of those characteristics. Indirect discrimination is said to occur when there are policies or rules that apply to all yet deemed unfair to those who share an attribute that "protects" a person with definable characteristics with the label "disabled" being applied. The Assistance Dog then becomes an extension of that person. Yet both direct and indirect discrimination against those who utilise Assistance Dogs is a growing issue and potentially underreported. Nevertheless, discrimination can have devastating effects such as worsening of symptoms (Vargas et al., 2020), emotional distress (Tyerman et al., 2021), poor health outcomes (Vargas et al., 2020), and heightened negative public attitudes (Rodriguez et al., 2020; Ross et al., 2019).

For students who are handlers of assistance animals, arguably their stress has already begun, whose personal privacy has been invaded, and having been "outed" by the presence of their Assistance Dog upon stepping onto campus. Required to disclose the nature of their disabling condition, they have *potentially* been subjected to a risk assessment by Human Resources before classes have begun. Moreover, they have likely been subjected to non-inclusive language and quite possibly have been unable to find the applicable policy related to them. To emphasise these potential concerns, at some universities, Assistance Dog policies may not even comply with relevant laws. For those with disabling condition/s and already facing their own struggles, they have nevertheless had to complete extra documentation and also attended additional appointments with health care professionals should they wish to disclose to their institution. This can mean that students who require an Assistance Dog enter university enduring a more complicated process than many other enrolling students.

Universities can consider such circumstances, and the fact that being welcomed at university can have a big impact during the admission stage, particularly for those that may have faced discrimination in the past (Sánchez-Herrero et al., 2021). This means that universities now need to help both handlers and

Assistance Dogs to successfully integrate, and this is where educative measures are vital. Universities should support handlers and their animals to ensure they do not enter classes where other students and staff are also perhaps ill-informed or uneducated as to the relevant legislation surrounding Assistance Dogs. If this does not occur, stigma, stereotyping, and negative public perceptions can be a very real outcome for the student (Nieforth et al., 2022; Rodriguez et al., 2019).

Stigma and stereotyping in educational settings can affect students' mental health and wellbeing. "Stigma is a socially constructed mark of disapproval, shame or disgrace that causes significant disadvantage through the curtailment of opportunities" (Martin, 2010, p. 261), and it deprives one of their dignity while also disrupting social harmony (Das, 2020). For people with a disabling condition, the fear of being excluded may contribute to them not appropriately responding their disability status upon enrolment into universities However, having an Assistance Dog at their side places the student centrally at risk of social exclusion, stigmatisation, which may impact on their health and wellbeing (Rodriguez et al., 2020).

INCLUDE ME, INCLUDE MY DOG

There remains a lack of understanding related to what Assistance Dogs "do" for their Handlers. Oftentimes it is left to the Handler to explain what their Assistance Dog does for them, yet to ask a Handler may require them to inadvertently disclose the nature of their disabling condition (Nieforth et al., 2022). In Froling's seminal work (2009), she cites many examples of activities that Assistance Dogs are trained to do in order to alleviate the symptoms of the handler's condition/s. While most handlers have been well-versed in these tasks and their Assistance Dogs individually trained, it is important for all university staff to have a basic understanding of a range of tasks Assistance Dogs can do. This gives the student's lecturer, professor, or tutor, an opportunity to demonstrate their commitment to creating an *inclusive* environment and show awareness and understanding by going the extra step by educating oneself about Assistance Dogs.

Inclusiveness can be demonstrated by understanding that Assistance Dogs are trained for many tasks and perform these in the public arena for their Handlers. In addition, they also have needs of their own (generally perhaps to change position or require to toilet). A certain amount of leeway should be provided for the student with the Assistance Dog, such as adequate seating arrangements so the Assistance Dog has room to move comfortably at the base of the foot well in class, social distancing is observed and no engagement with the Assistance Dog should be the rule. So, if the student and Assistance Dog need to leave class, it is important not to identify them and ask them a reason. This is unnecessary and arguably discriminatory as they are being singled out (Hopkins, 2011). There will be most likely a very clear reason for them to leave and it is a private matter.

Other barriers that have been further highlighted since the COVID-19 pandemic require further examination. The Assistance Dog is a source of attention, approached for a pat while working, and the requirement, and difficulty, for social distancing are faced daily. The advent of the pandemic highlighted these concerns of handlers in a way that engendered fear, and in some cases, became the impetus behind a movement that prompted handlers to stay within the safety of their home, rather than deal with these public interactions (which could have very real consequences to themselves and their dogs). Being asked to pat their Assistance Dog not only meant a (potential) refusal by the Handler, but also, required one to break government mandated social distancing requirements, notwithstanding the possible transmission of COVID-19. Throughout the pandemic, there were concerns about transmission from person to Assistance Dog, but also, zoonotic transmission that may occur from Assistance Dog to person or, person to Assistance Dog. This type of transmission has now been addressed by the Centres for Disease Control and Prevention (CDC) (2021). Within the CDC recommendations include remaining 6 feet (1.5 metres) away from others, not taking your Assistance Dog where others are infected with COVID-19 and regularly cleaning collars, vests and leashes to avoid transmission of this virus (Centres for Disease Control and Prevention, 2021). Assistance Dog Handlers have further concerns if their animal were to become infected with COVID-19. However, there remains an absence on advice in Australia on how to treat a possibly COVID-19 positive dog, but also, given handlers may be immunocompromised themselves, risk possible transmission and far-reaching health consequences to the handler.

FROM STIGMA TO EMPOWERMENT: CREATING A PRODUCTIVE ENVIRONMENT

From the perspective of being an Assistance Dog Handler, there are many ways to gain, re-gain, and maintain empowerment. First and foremost, it is vital to be cognisant of the legislation, maintain contact with Disability Services at the university, know the Policies of the University and *do not hesitate to challenge them* if they are incorrect. There are also many advocates that can be utilised should you feel you need support by your side (for example university disability services, equal opportunity, or supportive members of the faculty) (Grimes et al., 2020). Ensure that you have a healthcare team that excel at what they do and are supportive of you and your chosen treatment modality using an Assistance Dog. They can also be a great source of support and can also empower you along the way.

Issues such as being refused entry, singled out, being a source of attention and being asked to pat your Assistance Dog are only some of a myriad of areas that the student will come across. The lecturer of a client asked the Assistance Dog to remain outside a classroom tethered to a tree during a tutorial. As such it is vital that you are prepared to deal with these issues as they arise, and the university should implement regular inclusive training that includes students with Assistance Dogs and the legislation surrounding this—supporting the student and being aware of the legislation is imperative.

Handlers do need to take the responsibility to educate both the university and students of the potential consequences of their working dog; however, *they are not obliged to divulge the nature of their disability* to everyone (Human Rights Commission, 2016). What may be useful is to sit down with a mentor or Canine Behaviourist and develop a strategy prior to entering the university arena. Most often, Assistance Dog Handlers have cards made up that explain what Assistance Dogs do, the legislation in dot point form, and requests not to pat the dog. It is prudent that the public be informed of the gravity of the situation and what distraction can mean for the owner (Health Direct Australia, 2020). Thus, if you don't want to talk about your Assistance Dog, a card is oftentimes a great way to deflect and move on (Please Don't Pat Me Australia, 2022). This should also be addressed immediately by Disability Services and we would recommend they implement classes that educate all students and staff about Assistance Dogs and what they do to negate the singling out and stereotyping that can occur (Guide Dogs Australia, 2022). From the university's point of view, assigned role models (Swinburne University, 2022), pioneers or advocates may fill this critical gap (Human Rights Commission, 2021). Should dedicated role models be assigned (e.g., a professional that leads by example), they can then become knowledgeable about the situations faced by students with Assistance Dogs (Swinburne University, 2022). This can be a wonderful opportunity for them to take the role of advocate and assist students to become firmer or, take this role on themselves, in whichever manner this may be.

Assistance Dogs can be used for any number of reasons such as medication retrieval, hypoglycaemic events, combating emotional overloads (such as nudging or whining), cover to prevent panic attacks, alert for seizures, and to provide speech impairment assistance by carrying notes to specific people by using hand commands (Froling, 2009; Hardin et al., 2015) Being a source of attention and being asked to pat your dog can be contentious issue for handlers and where the development of strategies comes into play. Perhaps social distance mandates and consideration of potential toxicity of hand sanitiser (Stice et al., 2018) related to patting and the Assistance Dog should be pointed out by Handler, advocate or role model. Handlers should expect immediate compliance by the public given these core aspects have very real consequences to both handler (in terms of COVID-19 transmission) and Assistance Dog (potential toxicity from alcohol-based preparations (Stice et al., 2018) and COVID-19 transmission to the animal (Centres for Disease Control and Prevention, 2022)).

INCLUSIVENESS: ACCOMMODATE OUR NEEDS PLEASE!

We consider from our shared experience that tensions have heightened during the effects of the global COVID-19 pandemic. Assistance Dogs may have deskilled with the lockdowns that occurred during 2020–2022. Handlers need to reskill their Assistance Dogs in a safe space. They also need levels of understanding from those in positions of "power" to understand this space and to recognise the further pressures the pandemic placed on us all as a team (Abat-Roy, 2020).

To that end, the COVID-19 testing university mandates and the subsequent fear of hotel quarantines which have raised anxiety levels (Pratt & Tolkach, 2022; Rosen et al., 2020). These quarantines did not accommodate Assistance Dogs and in many cases prompted the handler to stay home rather than risk catching COVID-19 (Almendros, 2020; Centres for Disease Control and Prevention, 2021; Jezierski et al., 2021). These (realised or unrealised) fears arguably became a cycle of the Assistance Dog further deskilling as avoidance of public spaces occurred and the Assistance Dog was not "worked" as usual in public spaces (Jezierski et al., 2021). Yet these fears have been alleviated with the movement towards an online teaching and learning environment. The ability to study and work from home has allowed the mitigation of some anxiety in ourselves, and notably, others seeing the Assistance Dog who is often off duty at home has been a point of social connection during a period of social isolation. There have been many online teaching sessions that started out with engagement with the off-duty Assistance Dogs that then promoted connection with others onscreen.

However, despite the positive online presence of the Assistance Dog, Assistance Dog Handlers are also required to juggle the inevitable "bark" by Assistance Dogs who think they are "off the clock" and not in public—so there is still some navigation of the home environment and modification of the dog's "home" behaviours while attending university in an online capacity.

Teaching and learning have evolved post-pandemic. Thus, the need for a balance approach is required, given that continuance of blended teaching and learning in university environments. While this has allowed greater accessibility for many students to access teaching materials, it has potential to expand social connections and also provided a number of job opportunities. There are also other challenges that need to be navigated. The balance between teaching and learning in a home environment with an Assistance Dog "not working" and being "just dogs" has not been considered in a policy context. For example, during lockdowns there were university expectations to attend meetings online or teach at allocated times, without consideration of the Assistance Dog needs. Time must be allocated (regardless of commitments in the university) to use good weather to toilet Assistance Dogs during rainy days and make use of opportune times to exercise them (and the handlers too, to ensure our mental health needs are met). This "new space" that has not been supported by the university schedule.

DISCRIMINATION AND CONSEQUENCES

Awareness need to be raised and negative attitudes challenged in order to create a more accessible environment for persons who have disabling conditions (Brown & Leigh, 2018). This is critical because of the prejudicial attitudes and stigmatisation that frequently occur (Krnjacki et al., 2018), and the disability bias that still exists (Brown & Leigh, 2018). Evidence clearly remains that the consequences for those who have disabling condition/s include barriers to adjustments, prevention of social integration, being labelled and "a loss of status based on power differentials" (Brown & Leigh, 2018; Coleman et al., 2015). This is comparable to the findings of Krnjacki et al. (2018), who found that disability-based discrimination is a key determinant of poorer health outcomes. As such, the physical and emotional outcomes for the individual can be devastating (Brown & Leigh, 2018; Coleman et al., 2015).

That said, if people approach a person with an Assistance Dog in a positive manner, there are significant positive gains that can be made, both in the person's self-esteem, community integration and psychological wellbeing (Ross et al., 2019). Conversely, the attention can cause negative reactions, engendering feelings of invasion of personal space (inclusive of social distancing requirements) (Ratschen et al., 2020), increased visibility of disablement, and amplifying stigma that could have been avoided without the presence of an Assistance Dog (Das, 2020; Tyerman et al., 2021).

The time taken for unnecessary assessments, risk assessments, the utilisation of other departments such as Human Resources, and sustained silence by the universities post-pandemic all has a cost. As such, it would be beneficial for universities to implement programs that would positively improve students' lives and their health and wellbeing. For this to happen, students must remain empowered throughout the university experience, and universities need to make reasonable adjustments as outlined throughout this chapter. If universities seek advice from experienced Canine Behaviourists/Psychologists cognisant with the legal aspects and "going the extra mile", this can indeed be negated *without undue hardship*.

CONCLUSION

All universities should consider their policies and training in relation to Assistance Dogs on campus to ensure they comply with national laws. Universities should also consider the current conditions that Assistance Dog Handlers exist in, with the risk of COVID infection remaining and the challenge of handling a dog throughout this situation and into the future. Policies developed and uploaded to university websites is simply not enough. These need to be complied with and embedded in the culture of universities, from administrative staff, to lecturers, to Deans, to Professors, all the way up to the Vice Chancellor. Policies need to be amended (if they exist) and subsequently should be a lived example to ensure that stigma, stereotyping and exclusionary practices are stamped out and inclusionary practices are embedded in curricula so unnecessary assessment remains a thing of the past. Universities have a responsibility to protect the mental health of their students from stigma and stereotyping. The presence of an Assistance Dog essentially 'outs' the student and places them at greater risk—more so if the university has a disability risk management policy in place. Universities need to have in place protective mechanisms for the student and arguably a more structured support network than is often in place to support at risk students. For only then, can student who utilise Assistance Dogs as a treatment modality, mobility aid and so on will flourish in their university experience, achieve greatness, and succeed in their studies.

REFERENCES

Abat-Roy, V. (2020, July 10). COVID-19 presents new obstacles for people who use service dogs. *The Conversation*. https://theconversation.com/covid-19-presents-new-obstacles-for-people-who-use-service-dogs-141965

Almendros, A. (2020). Can companion animals become infected with COVID-19? *The Veterinary Record, 186*(12), 388. https://doi.org/https://doi.org/10.1136/vr.m1194

Brown, N., & Leigh, J. (2018). Ableism in academia: Where are the disabled and ill academics? *Disability & Society, 33*(6), 985–989.

Centres for Disease Control and Prevention. (2021). *Guidance for handlers of service and therapy animals*. Centres for Disease Control and Prevention. Retrieved April 25, 2022, from https://stacks.cdc.gov/view/cdc/88829

Centres for Disease Control and Prevention. (2022). *Animals and COVID-19*. Centres for Disease Control and Prevention. Retrieved May 1, 2022, from https://www.cdc.gov/coronavirus/2019-ncov/daily-life-coping/animals.html

Coleman, J. A., Ingram, K. M., Bays, A., Joy-Gaba, J. A., & Boone, E. L. (2015). Disability and assistance dog implicit association test: a novel IAT. *Rehabilitation Psychology, 60*(1), 17–26.

Commonwealth of Australia. (1992). *Disability Discrimination Act*. Australian Federal Government. Retrieved February 14, 2017, from http://www.austlii.edu.au/au/legis/cth/consol_act/dda1992264/

Das, M. (2020). Social construction of stigma and its implications–observations from COVID-19. *Social Sciences and Humanities, Pre Print*, 1–27. Retrieved May 1, 2022, from https://papers.ssrn.com/sol3/Delivery.cfm/7d4ae588-d46e-4582-be1b-b04b35c3034c-MECA.pdf?abstractid=3599764&mirid=1

Equality and Human Rights Commission. (2018). *Home page*. Equality and Human Rights Commission. Retrieved April 25, 2018, from https://www.equalityhumanrights.com/en

Froling, J. (2009). *Service dog tasks for psychiatric disabilities*. Sterling Service Dogs. Retrieved 9 April 2018 from http://www.iaadp.org/psd_tasks.html

Geller, G. (2018). *What is an assistance dog*. Canine Essentials Pty. Ltd. Retrieved March 13, 2018, from http://www.canineessentials.com.au/about-assistance-dogs/

Government of NSW. (1977). *Anti-Discrimination Act 1977 No 48*. https://legislation.nsw.gov.au/view/whole/html/inforce/current/act-1977-048

Government of South Australia. (1984). *Equal Opportunity Act*. Government of South Australia. Retrieved February 14, 2017, from https://www.legislation.sa.gov.au/LZ/C/A/Equal%20Opportunity%20Act%201984.aspx

Gravrok, J., Howell, T., Bendrups, D., & Bennett, P. (2019). Thriving through Relationships: Assistance dogs' and companion dogs' perceived ability to contribute to thriving in individuals with and without a disability. *Disability and Rehabilitation: Assistive Technology*.

Grimes, S., Southgate, E., Scevak, J., & Buchanan, R. (2020). University student experiences of disability and the influence of stigma on institutional non-disclosure and learning. *Journal of Postsecondary Education and Disability*, 33(1), 23–37.

Guide Dogs Australia. (2022). *Advocacy: Systemic and Individual*. Guide Dogs Australia. Retrieved April 15, 2022, from https://guidedogs.com.au/get-support/making-the-world-more-accessible/systemic-and-individual-advocacy/#about-our-advocacy-partners

Hardin, D. S., Anderson, W., & Cattet, J. (2015). Dogs can be successfully trained to alert to hypoglycemia samples from patients with type 1 diabetes. *Diabetes Therapy*, 6(4), 509–517.

Health Direct Australia. (2020). *Assistance dogs*. Health Direct Australia. Retrieved April 1, 2022, from https://www.healthdirect.gov.au/assistance-dogs

Hopkins, L. (2011). The path of least resistance: A voice-relational analysis of disabled students' experiences of discrimination in English universities. *International Journal of Inclusive Education*, 15(7), 711–727.

Human Rights Commission. (2016). *Assistance animals and the Disability Discrimination Act 1992 (Cth)*. Human Rights Commission. https://www.humanrights.gov.au/our-work/disability-rights/projects/assistance-animals-and-disability-discrimination-act-1992-cth

Human Rights Commission. (2021). *Disability action plan guide (2021)*. Human Rights Commission. Retrieved April 15, 2022, from https://humanrights.gov.au/sites/default/files/document/publication/ahrc_disability_action_plan_guide_2021_0.pdf

Jezierski, T., Camerlink, I., Peden, R. S. E., Chou, J.-Y., & Marchewka, J. (2021, August 1). Changes in the health and behaviour of pet dogs during the COVID-19 pandemic as reported by the owners. *Applied Animal Behaviour Science*, 241, 1–8. https://doi.org/https://doi.org/10.1016/j.applanim.2021.105395

Krnjacki, L., Priest, N., Aitken, Z., Emerson, E., Llewellyn, G., King, T., & Kavanagh, A. (2018). Disability-based discrimination and health: findings from an Australian-based population study. *Australian and New Zealand Journal of Public Health, 42*(2), 172–174.

Martin, J. M. (2010). Stigma and student mental health in higher education. *Higher Education Research & Development, 29*(3), 259–274.

Nieforth, L. O., Rodriguez, K. E., & O'Haire, M. E. (2022). Expectations versus experiences of veterans with posttraumatic stress disorder (PTSD) service dogs: An inductive conventional content analysis. *Psychological Trauma: Theory, Research, Practice, and Policy, 14*(3), 1–10.

Pratt, S., & Tolkach, D. (2022). Affective and coping responses to quarantine hotel stays. *Stress and Health, Early View*(n/a). https://doi.org/https://doi.org/10.1002/smi.3126

Ratschen, E., Shoesmith, E., Shahab, L., Silva, K., Kale, D., Toner, P., Reeve, C., & Mills, D. S. (2020). Human-animal relationships and interactions during the COVID-19 lockdown phase in the UK: Investigating links with mental health and loneliness. *PloS One, 15*(9), e0239397.

Rodriguez, K. E., Bibbo, J., Verdon, S., & O'Haire, M. E. (2019). Mobility and medical service dogs: A qualitative analysis of expectations and experiences. *Disability and Rehabilitation: Assistive Technology*.

Rodriguez, K. E., Bibbo, J., Verdon, S., & O'Haire, M. E. (2020, July 3). Mobility and medical service dogs: a qualitative analysis of expectations and experiences. *Disability and Rehabilitation: Assistive Technology, 15*(5), 499–509. https://doi.org/10.1080/17483107.2019.1587015

Rosen, Z., Weinberger-Litman, S. L., Rosenzweig, C., Rosmarin, D. H., Muennig, P., Carmody, E. R., Rao, S. T., & Litman, L. (2020). Anxiety and distress among the first community quarantined in the US due to COVID-19: Psychological implications for the unfolding crisis. *PrePrint*, 1–18. https://doi.org/10.31234/osf.io/7eq8c

Ross, A. M., Morgan, A. J., Jorm, A. F., & Reavley, N. J. (2019). A systematic review of the impact of media reports of severe mental illness on stigma and discrimination, and interventions that aim to mitigate any adverse impact. *Social Psychiatry and Psychiatric Epidemiology, 54*(1), 11–31.

Sánchez-Herrero, H., Amezcua-Prieto, C., Morales-Suárez-Varela, M., Ayán-Pérez, C., Mateos-Campos, R., Molina, A. J., Ortiz-Moncada, R., Almaraz-Gómez, A., Alguacil, J., Delgado-Rodríguez, M., Blázquez Abellán, G., Alonso-Molero, J., Martínez-Ruiz, V., Peraita-Costa, I., Cancela-Carral, J. M., Valero-Juan, L. F., Martín-Peláez, S., & Fernández-Villa, T. (2021). Discrimination and its relationship with risk behaviors and perceived health in Spanish university students: A cross-sectional study. *Revista espanola de salud publica, 95*, e202111156. Retrieved 2021/11, from http://europepmc.org/abstract/MED/34779425

Stice, S., Thrall, M. A., & Hamar, D. W. (2018). Chapter 49 - Alcohols and Glycols. In R. C. Gupta (Ed.), *Veterinary toxicology* (3rd ed., pp. 647–657). Academic Press. https://doi.org/https://doi.org/10.1016/B978-0-12-811410-0.00049-0

Swinburne University. (2022). *Swinburne international alum inspiring change together with her guide dog Elke*. Swinburne University. Retrieved June 2, 2022, from https://www.swinburne.edu.au/news/2022/03/swinburne-international-alum-inspiring-change-together-with-her-with-her-guide-dog-elke/

Tsang, M. C. C., Bould, E., Lalor, A., & Callaway, L. (2021). 'Community members aren't aware that assistance animals come in all shapes and sizes, and help people with all kinds of disabilities'–Experiences of using assistance animals within community living in Australia. *Disability and Rehabilitation: Assistive Technology*, 1–11. https://doi.org/https://doi.org/10.1080/17483107.2021.1938709

Tyerman, J., Patovirta, A.-L., & Celestini, A. (2021, February 1). How stigma and discrimination influences nursing care of persons diagnosed with mental illness: A systematic review. *Issues in Mental Health Nursing, 42*(2), 153–163. https://doi.org/10.1080/01612840.2020.1789788

UK Government. (2010). *Equality Act*. UK Government. Retrieved April 24, 2018, from https://www.legislation.gov.uk/ukpga/2010/15/contents

U.S. Department of Justice: Civil Rights Division. (2017). *A guide to disability rights laws*. U.S. Department of Justice. Retrieved April 25, 2018, from https://www.ada.gov/cguide.htm

US Department of Justice. (2010). *Americans with Disabilities Act: Service animals*. US Department of Justice. Retrieved April 24, 2018, from https://www.ada.gov/service_animals_2010.htm

Vargas, S. M., Huey, S. J., & Miranda, J. (2020). A critical review of current evidence on multiple types of discrimination and mental health. *American journal of orthopsychiatry, 90*(3), 374–390. https://doi.org/10.1037/ort0000441

Victorian Equal Opportunity & Equal Rights Commission. (2017). *Australian human rights framework*. Victorian Equal Opportunity & Equal Rights Commission. Retrieved February 14, 2017, from https://www.humanrights.vic.gov.au/legal-and-policy/australias-human-rights-framework/

CHAPTER 15

Universalizing International Exchange for Students with Disabilities

JUSTIN HARFORD

INTRODUCTION

Evaluating a Title IX claim for gender-based discrimination on a South Africa-bound faculty lead exchange program in 2002, a US District Court in Michigan found that study abroad programs are an integral part of post-compulsory education today (King v. Board of Control of Eastern Michigan University, 2002). That court decision, nearly 20 years ago, was symptomatic of a trend in which studying or interning overseas was increasingly identified as an inseparable component of a college experience—so much so that a federal court was suggesting that failure to ensure international exchange was free of discrimination would be the same as failure to ensure a college education without discrimination. Since then, the connection between exchange and college has become even more acute. A growing body of research suggests a correlation between successful employment outcomes and certain kinds of international exchange (Richard et al., 2017). In order to have access to all the benefits of a college education, all students must be able to participate in international exchange.

Nevertheless, barriers continue to discourage the participation of underrepresented students in international exchange programs. LGBTQ, first-generation, ethnic minority, low-income and disabled students can get overwhelmed by the perceived costs, the logistical difficulties or the fear of being treated differently, and they can underestimate the resources available to them. A great deal of effort has been dedicated towards increasing the numbers of students participating through targeted recruitment, education or scholarships. A great deal more will be required to get more disabled students to study abroad, and essential step to achieve true inclusion.

This chapter reflects on why international exchange is so important for people with disabilities, the current state of the field, and how travelers with disabilities and exchange program staff can move it forward. The reader will take away a healthy dose of optimism about the future of students with disabilities in international exchange. This chapter provides a roadmap for bringing about a world where everyone can access international education regardless of their condition and regardless of the destination.

Through my study abroad in Chile, I experienced the realities and the potentials of international exchange as a blind person. I faced down what seemed like intractable challenges. I figured out how to show up as a newcomer to an unfamiliar campus. I accessed a rigorous course curriculum with 250 pages of Spanish language reading each week—without using a service to digitize the material. I traveled alone for a few weeks around neighboring countries.

While abroad, I also encountered different views of disability. Some were negative: I could be and was refused entry to places of public accommodation for being blind. In other cases, they were positive; such as the normality of asking for help in a culture which emphasized community and interdependence rather than individuality and independence. That made it easier to get help doing archival research.

International exchange boosted my confidence as a person with a disability, and through my time abroad I learned that I could accomplish many things if I put my mind to it. Since then I have searched for ways to increase the participation of people with disabilities in international exchange by advising and developing resources.

WHERE WE ARE AT

The idea of people with disabilities participating in international exchange programs is not new. Newel Perry was a blind mathematician who completed his Ph.D in Munich around the turn of the 20th century (Wittenstein, 2014). The Fulbright accepted its first disabled participant in 1955. Susan Sygall, the founder of Mobility International USA and a wheelchair user, earned her Master's degree in Australia with the support of the Rotary Peace Fellowship (PWAG, n.d.). Every year, people with disabilities from all walks of life study, volunteer or intern overseas. Exchange programs respond well to participants with disabilities and requests for reasonable accommodations. In certain cases, programs even would go above and beyond by doing direct outreach to the disability community (Ablaeva, 2012).

Colleges have made improvements at including people with disabilities, but there is still much more to be done. Many exchange programs still wait until someone with a disability applies before learning about the resources available (Ablaeva, 2012). As a result of this reactive approach, there is still a great degree of uncertainty for a disabled participant seeking to study abroad. Disability-specific information on overseas sites for accommodations like accessible housing, sign language interpreters or alternative media is limited or nonexistent. People with disabilities sometimes must rely on guidance from friends and family, which may be erroneous. Prospective exchange participants with disabilities sometimes find themselves in the role of managing doubts of the exchange staff rather than the other way around (Ablaeva, 2012). No wonder that many disabled people simply assume that international exchange is not an option for them (Holben & Ozel, 2015).

DESIGN ACCESS FROM THE GROUND UP

Exchange professionals share a variety of concerns about participants with disabilities. One of the most common relates to disclosure (Ablaeva, 2012). When prospective exchange participants don't disclose their conditions early on, it can be difficult for exchange professionals to make the necessary preparations. In other cases, the student may disclose, and the program is then faced with a situation that they had not prepared for when the program was first conceived. Last-minute scrambles for accessible housing or sign language interpreters fall neatly into this category.

Though these inquiries touch on a variety of topics, they are all linked to the underlying fact that exchange programs continue to be conceived, designed and renovated without considering the full breadth of prospective participants. Many exchange programs are attempting to engage with new diverse groups of students, while continuing to design their programs for the traditional groups that they had always served (Soneson & Cordano, 2009). In the case of participants with disabilities, this means that program organisers rush to retrofit housing, transportation and programmatic arrangements at the last minute, stressing out program organizers or unnecessarily excluding disabled participants. Since most of the issues of including people with disabilities in international exchange start with the way that programs are designed, the logical solution is to design the physical, academic, cultural, and programmatic arrangement to automatically receive the widest group of potential participants. Principles of universal design, originally developed for the field of architecture, should be applied to international exchange programs in the same way that they have been utilized in other areas of academia (Soneson & Cordano, 2009).

Program administrators need to focus on the things that are under their control and learn as much as possible about what is not. Are overseas partners aware of, and on board with, policies of disability inclusion? Can the program supply information that a prospective participant with disabilities would need to know when deciding whether and how to proceed? Are policies designed to work with participants with disabilities who experience setbacks? Are staff trained to implement those policies and to exercise basic cultural competence when working with people with disabilities? Do recruitment strategies communicate that people with disabilities are welcome by promoting positive images of people with disabilities successfully studying or interning overseas? If a building does not have an elevator, would all classes be held on the first floor? Are host families trained about disability culture, and is there at least one housing situation that could be made accessible? Finally, is the program able to meet people with a variety of reasonable accommodation needs, and varying levels of willingness to disclose without necessarily requiring disclosure for program staff to be comfortable?

SELECTING A PROGRAM

When a student examines a program, or when a program examines itself, the following questions must be considered: Can a program supply accessibility information about a host country? Are there disabled contacts with whom they could put a student in touch to learn about policies or facilities that disabled people use to go about daily life? Are there positive depictions of people with disabilities participating in overseas activities in program materials, including photos, videos and blogs? Is it possible to find information about how to request reasonable accommodations, counseling resources or links to organizations about travel and disability? Can recruiters answer disability-related questions? Do staff have a proactive can-do attitude about a students' goals?

Students with disabilities need to know as much as possible about a program of interest and how it relates to what they want to accomplish by the time they submit their application. While it can be tempting to select a program based on assumptions about its inclusion of people with disabilities, each student should challenge themselves to choose a program based on their personal, academic and professional aspirations. A location like Australia, England or Germany will offer more modern accessible amenities, but if the student wants to study Swahili, or research politics in East Asia, they would do better to go to a slightly less traditional place like Kenya or Mongolia. Each student needs to think about the ways that they adapt to their disability, identify adaptations they can take to a chosen destination, and consider alternatives for the rest.

What is meant by "alternatives?" The biggest support that I couldn't take overseas was the book digitalization service. My alternative was to scan books myself using photocopy machines, and to recruit volunteer readers. A wheelchair user might be accustomed to using public buses in the United States, but they might find that taxies are more effective for Mexico City. A student with diabetes might need to get an extra supply of insulin or learn where they can get it in a host country.

A student does not have to rely exclusively on their program to get what they need. I found support from the host university's engineering department, who lent me their scanner. This came to me after I met someone from the department as I was orienting myself to the campus. Chilean students, recruited from the school of humanities through flyer and email campaigns, spent hours reading to me. Friends from travel forums accompanied me to places I would not have been allowed to visit on my own. I would not have been able to predict that I would find these resources, but proactive problem-solving and thinking about ways that I could offer value to other people, such as through English tutoring, made all the difference. Even if a program says that something is "not possible," that does not mean that the student cannot make it possible by using alternative resources.

INFORMATION IS KEY

Institutions should have a good sense of the disability resources available at their host centers and partner sites around the world as a first step towards ironing out the wrinkles in their reasonable accommodation process. Some universities refer to their disability service offices and host partners to gather accessibility information about locations overseas. Many institutions have even posted accessibility-specific information on their websites, so a prospective student can get an idea of what their situation will look like in the host country. Ensuring that exchange advisors are broadly aware of resources, and where prospective participants can find them, will help ensure that both participants with disabilities and exchange staff are on the same page.

Institutions and students need to avoid limiting their interpretations of accessibility to wheelchair ramps and Braille materials. While those are certainly important, one can be tempted to overlook the reasonable accommodations required by people with other kinds of disabilities or the cultural alternatives that can stretch the notion of what is possible. A couple of strong peers or locals can enable a wheelchair user to get over a step. A network of professional copy centers can be a great alternative to alternative media. A video communication service like Skype or Google Hangouts can help a student continue meeting with their therapist while overseas. More affordable drug prices or nationalized healthcare can make medication and treatment easier to access. International exchange demands an expanded notion of accessibility for both exchange planners and participants. This can be achieved with the right information.

How is this information found? Exchange professionals have their networks including in-country hosts, university faculty, host country staff and alumni with disabilities. They can also identify host country Disabled People's Organizations. Students also have the option of reaching out to those sources, either through their study abroad program or their own efforts. The Disability Rights Education and Defense Fund (DREDF), for example, offers a guide to the disability rights laws of countries around the world. Students and staff can search around online to see what people connected with disability and higher education in the host country say about it on forums, blogs, radio or YouTube videos. Host country university faculty can tell you about accommodations that their students have received and their contact info can often be located on department web pages.

Each participant must take an active role in doing this research. Exchange staff cannot know exactly what someone's accommodation needs may be, nor can they know about the reasonable accommodations that work for the individual at their home campus, and the accommodations that they can and cannot be without. Programs should have a conversation about these questions with the participant, and the participant should already be in the process of finding the answers.

ACTIVE RECRUITMENT

Institutions must develop a recruitment strategy to attract people with disabilities. Without this, disabled people will not know that a program is accessible or that they are welcome to apply. Disability recruitment should be an integral part of program outreach. If the institution has an Accessibility Resource Center, they will be an ideal partner. Such centers can help get the word out about study abroad fairs or panels, and programs can even send staff to meet directly with students with disabilities.

Recruitment materials should always be made in multiple and accessible formats. A student should be able to log onto an institution's exchange programs website and view stories, photos or videos of people participating in the programs, visually and through audio description. Those depictions might include people using wheelchairs, canes or other adaptive devices, demonstrating the institution's commitment and desire to welcome all. Include disability in the nondiscrimination statement if it isn't already. In time, disabled alumni of programs will present to other peers with disabilities about how they benefited from their times abroad with an institution's program.

INFILTRATION

If you are a student, don't wait for an invitation to a study abroad program. International exchange is one of the most formative experiences that you will have in college, and it would be unfortunate to lose such an opportunity simply because the program wasn't ready for you. While you cannot be sure of having the most flawless experience when you are trailblazing, it certainly has its unique rewards. I can't remember many other experiences in my life where I was so fully in charge of a project and where I expanded my conception of my own abilities.

It takes courage. As a student, you could be placing a lot in the balance, from course credit to financial aid, without much certainty of even the basics, such as the supports that you have relied on at your home campus. But everything worth having involves risk, and when people around you see what you are trying to do, they will rally to your aid. Stories can be an extremely helpful motivating factor. Mobility International USA and Abroad with Disabilities regularly post success stories of people with different kinds of disabilities volunteering and studying overseas. Peruse those materials to get an idea of what is possible. Consider sharing your own story when you get back.

CONCLUSION

International exchange is becoming an even more integral part of higher education. Seeing nondisabled peers going overseas will urge disabled students to ask for similar opportunities. Perceptions of a changing legal landscape will also raise their expectations. We have already seen this with the Americans with Disabilities Act (ADA), which has led American students with disabilities to presume an increasingly wider range of rights in higher education (Rothstein, 2008). There has also been a proliferation of disability rights legislation in over 180 countries (Shapiro, 2015). That may result in a similarly expanded notion of rights among disabled people around the world. It does not seem like much of a stretch to suppose that people with disabilities will begin to expect full access, both at home and overseas.

Exchange administrators should not wait for the first application to begin planning for access. By working with their partners to figure out what is available at host sites, they will not only be able to inform themselves, but also prospective applicants with disabilities. By publishing stories and testimonies on the website, along with positive depictions of disabled participants overseas, the overseas program will send a clear message that everyone is welcome. By incorporating discussions of mental health, and reasonable accommodations in orientation materials for participants and staff, such programs can lead by example, and demonstrate a commitment to increased participation.

For prospective participants with disabilities looking to go on their first, or even their second or third international exchange, the bigger their dreams the better. Talk with fellow disabled students. Consult a program's website. Meet with an advisor to get a sense of what can be expected in the way of collaboration from the program. Reach out to organizations in the host country including university faculty, people with disabilities, service providers and travel companies. Embrace the risk. International exchange is such a formative and valuable experience.

Whether you are staff or student, remember that you are in this together. Each party is an important resource for the other. The collaboration will be most effective with open communication and information sharing. A student will enhance their ability to negotiate and strategize for their own success in a way that pragmatically considers competing interests, while not settling for less. Staff will develop tools for including diverse students, while learning more inclusive ways of working. Both should make sure that at the end of the day, they each can tell a story of success that they can be proud of, and lessons that they can build on for the future.

REFERENCES

Ablaeva, Y. S. (2012). *Inclusion of students with disabilities in study abroad: Current practices and student perspectives* (Unpublished master's thesis). University of Oregon, Eugene, Oregon. Retrieved from https://scholarsbank.uoregon.edu/xmlui/bitstream/handle/1794/12426/Ablaeva_oregon_0171N_10417.pdf?sequence=1

Bureau of Educational and Cultural Affairs. (n.d.). *Disability and international exchange programs timeline*. United States Department of State. Retrieved from https://eca.state.gov/video/disability-international-exchange-programs-timeline/transcript

Holben, A., & Ozel, C. (2015). International exchange with a disability: Enhancing experiences abroad through advising and mentoring. *Journal of Postsecondary Education and Disability, 28*(4), 405–412. Retrieved from https://files.eric.ed.gov/fulltext/EJ1093584.pdf

King v. Board of Control of Eastern Michigan University 221 F. Supp. 2d 783 (E.D. Mich. 2002) Retrieved from https://law.justia.com/cases/federal/district-courts/FSupp2/221/783/2486385/

Mobility International USA (MIUSA). (n.d.). *Disclosure and building trust*. Retrieved from http://www.miusa.org/resource/tipsheet/buildingtrust

Mobility International USA (MIUSA). (n.d.). *Students with disabilities and education abroad statistics*. Retrieved from http://www.miusa.org/resource/tipsheet/USstudentsatisfaction

Peace Women across the Globe (PWAG). (n.d.). *Susan Sygall, (United States of America)*. Retrieved from http://wikipeacewomen.org/wpworg/en/?page_id=3735

Prohn, S. M., Kelley, K. R., & Westling, D. L. (2015). Studying abroad inclusively: Reflections by college students with and without intellectual disability. *Journal of Intellectual Disabilities*, *20*(4), 341–353. Retrieved from https://files.eric.ed.gov/fulltext/EJ1123663.pdf

Richard, N., Lowe, R., & Hanks, C. (2017). *Gone international: Mobility works, report on the 2014–15 graduating cohort.* London, UK: UUKi. Retrieved from http://www.universitiesuk.ac.uk/policy-and-analysis/reports/Documents/International/GoneInternational2017_A4.pdf

Rothstein, L. (2008). Millennial's and disability law: Revisiting Southeastern Community College v. Davis. *Journal of College and University Law*, *34*(1), 1–29. Retrieved from https://ssrn.com/abstract=1266333

Shapiro, J. (2015, July 24). How a law to protect disabled Americans became imitated around the world. *National Public Radio*. Retrieved from https://www.npr.org/sections/goatsandsoda/2015/07/24/425607389/how-a-law-to-protect-disabled-americans-became-imitated-around-the-world

Soneson, H., & Cordano, R. J. (2009). Universal design and study abroad. *Frontiers: The Interdisciplinary Journal of Study Abroad*, 269–288. Retrieved from https://files.eric.ed.gov/fulltext/EJ883703.pdf

Wittenstein, S. (2014). *Newel Perry inducted 2014.* Retrieved from https://sites.aph.org/hall/inductees/perry/

CHAPTER 16

Creating an Accessible and Resilient Environment Inside the Indian University

P. BOOPATHI AND K. MURUGANANDAN

INTRODUCTION

In 1972, students passing out from Andha Mahavidyalaya higher secondary school for the blind began a sustained struggle for getting admitted to higher education by the Delhi University. One of the students started a hunger strike in front of then Prime Minister Indira Gandhi's residence. Subsequent struggles by blind organisations and blind students in colleges resulted in facilities such as tape recorders, braille books, readers, hostel accommodation and admission to professional courses from the University (Chander, 2008). This example and subsequent victories in the realm of disabled education illustrate that whatever accommodations and provisions have been provided to disabled students in higher education in India, they have been won over by hard struggles and through international pressures.

Lobbying by disabled students is a major force of change, however, creating environment for the disabled in Indian universities requires a lot more initiatives. A unique scheme to be paid special attention in this chapter is the scheme for the Higher Education for Persons with Special Needs (HEPSN) formulated by the University Grants Commission (UGC). This comprehensive scheme for the disabled in higher education is remarkable in three ways: Firstly, "Enabling Units" were encouraged to be established in colleges and universities for facilitating admission, providing guidance and counselling, and finding employment for the disabled students. HEPSN scheme introduced provisions for financial grants towards making colleges and universities infrastructurally and architecturally accessible for the disabled students. Finally, HEPSN scheme also granted allowances to provide special equipment for ensuring the delivery of better education with equal opportunity and easy access (University Grants Commission, 2008a).

Unfortunately, the HEPSN scheme has barely yielded the expected results. Many universities have not opened their centres; most of the universities administered by the state governments remain oblivious to any centre or provision for the disabled, as betrayed by their websites and policy documents. We could often hear from the coordinators of the available HEPSN units and Cell for the Disabled how financial difficulties are used to justify the absence of disability services to students. Common experiences of disabled students and faculty remain that most often than not, universities do not give due importance to the HEPSN Centre, as they consider it as an extra administrative as well as financial burden. Universities instead focus more on changing the name of the centre with well-coloured euphemisms like "differently abled" Centre/Office, and other patronising labels, rather than providing the students with conducive and accessible learning environment.

This chapter is a manifesto for change. It outlines clearly what needs to be done to make the aspirations of legislation and the promise of HEPSN unit a reality. In the US, 10.9% of the student population in higher education identifies as disabled (National Center for Education Statistics, 2016). In India, the number is 0.56%--less than 1% of India's 2.21 million students (Bansal, 2016). A lot remains to be done to improve the access of higher education for the disabled students in the Indian scenario.

In this chapter, we propose the strengthening of HEPSN Unit and the formation of a Central Committee for enhancing disability services and improving the living conditions of the disabled on university campuses. Much more can also be achieved with the formation of separate committees at each wing of the university and call for services and facilities both in the local and centralised manner by effective harnessing of available resources. This chapter provides clear-cut suggestions for achieving these institutional mechanisms and support systems for orienting universities disabled friendly. This chapter presents a blueprint for change, for closing the gap between rhetoric and reality.

DISABLED STUDENTS IN INDIAN HIGHER EDUCATION

India has an estimated 2.21% of the population identifying as disabled. According to the 2011 census, the literacy rate of those identifying as disabled was 54.5%, against an overall literacy rate of 74% (Bansal, 2016). Only 0.56% of the disabled population enrol for higher education some estimates suggest that not even 1% of Indian higher educational institutions are equipped with accessible campuses, classrooms,, teaching-learning materials and technologies for the disabled students, and many of them are characterised by hostile atmosphere against the disability conditions (Hindustan Times, 2017; Jameel, 2011; Saksena & Sharma, 2015).

University education, still a distant dream for a majority of Indians, is not able to include the disabled despite the enactment of several legislations and formulation of policies. Disabled students aspiring to enter higher education must hence cope with high poverty rates, lack of awareness among the general population, and the location of universities far from their homes. Additionally, many government funded universities have not even implemented the 5% reservation for the disabled in admission to the higher educational institutions ensured by the RPD Act, while private universities are not covered within the ambit of disability legislation (Shahi, 2016).

There exists a wide-spread administrative apathy, attitudinal bias and strongly entrenched stigma in universities that grossly affect the academic performances of disabled students (Jameel, 2011; Shahi, 2016). These prejudices and stereotypes play a crucial role in constructing the popular notion of disabled students as dependent and always in need of sympathy. However, lacking conducive learning environments, unavailability of course-materials in accessible format and barriers in accessing the library, residential places, canteens and other public places together combine to exclude disabled students from mainstream university activities.

In India, caste and poverty play out as additional impediments to accessible education, particularly in the post-school sector (Gabel & Danforth, 2008; University Grants Commission, 2008b). Gender, locality (urban versus rural), and cultural practices also contribute to these hurdles (Tilak, 2015). Disability, in combination with one or more of these factors, makes access even more difficult (Mehrotra, 2013).

CENTRAL COMMITTEE AND DISABILITY SERVICES: A MANIFESTO

The HEPSN Centre was mandated during the ninth five year plan (1997–2002) by UGC in all universities to create an accessible and barrier-free environment. The aim of establishing this centre was also to provide accessible technologies and course materials to disabled students (University Grants Commission, 2008b). Lack of financial support, coupled with a lack of awareness among university administrators, resulted in the scheme not yielding expected outcomes. For the reforms mandated by the University Grants Commission to be effective, universities must mainstream the HEPSN Unit and credit it with enough funding and full administrative support so as to increase the participation of disabled students in universities.

Universities do not pay enough attention to the HEPSN Centre and consider it as an extra burden for their day-today functioning. They need to revamp their HEPSN units and integrate these to their core administration to create accessible and inclusive environments for disabled students. This will help universities change their charity/sympathetic attitude towards the disabled to one of equity and inclusion. This integration will also make universities realize their responsibilities towards disabled students in creating accessible learning environments, barrier-free mobility inside campuses, and equal opportunities. The HEPSN Centre should be bestowed with the power to coordinate with other units like Women's Cell, Dean Students Welfare (DSW) Office, Student Unions, Equal Opportunity Cells, Administration, hostel committees and various schools/faculties. With the help of administration, the HEPSN Centre should form the Central Committee as a coordinating agency among all such units to look into the issues of disabled students in admission, teaching, learning, curriculum and examination, administration, campus environments, residence, transport, architecture and placement.

The coordinator of HEPSN Centre should be appointed as the chairman of the committee, for he/she is aware of issues faced by disabled students in all such aspects of university. As establishing HEPSN Centre and other mentioned units have been mandated by the UGC in all universities to address the problems faced by students from various religious, social, economic and cultural backgrounds, the HEPSN Centre should well coordinate with those units to represent and resolve the issues emanating from intersections such as religion, region, class, caste, gender and culture among disabled students. Understanding these intersections is very important, for most disabled students come from poor-economic backgrounds, rural areas and lower-caste families. Also, universities should be mindful of women disabled students, whose enrolment ratio is around 30–40% less than male disabled students (Jameel, 2011; Saksena & Sharma, 2015). Similarly, disabled students hailing from religious minority backgrounds should be given more attention by universities, as they tent to feel isolated both among their disabled peers and among their non-disabled associates. To address the issues emerging out of these intersections, universities should have one representative from each mentioned unit in the Central Committee. This will resolve the discrimination and exclusion faced by disabled students on top of their disability related challenges. Likewise, representatives from each school should also be appointed as a member of central committee to take up the issues pertaining to disabled students in particular schools.

Having the Central Committee as the coordinating and supervising body in disability related issues and policies, universities should set up school level committees to address the issues of disabled students within particular schools. In such committees, a representative from each departmental committee should be included. The dean of the school or a senior disabled faculty should be appointed as the chairperson of the school level committee. Each department should be asked to form departmental committees of 3 to 5 members to take care of the problems faced by disabled students within particular departments. The head of the committee can be the chairperson of the department or the disabled faculty serving in the department. The school level committee will coordinate and supervise the departmental committees to provide better learning environments and attend to the various needs and issues of disabled students.

The HEPSN Unit should be given enough funding to create a resource centre replete with accessible computers, Braille printer, snap-shot scanners, motorized wheelchairs, sign-language interpreters, hearing aids, etc. This resource centre should be under the direct supervision of HEPSN Units. Also, universities should allocate 5% of fund to the unit out of their annual funding from UGC as per the recently legislated RPD Act 2016. Besides setting up of resource centre to cater to the varied needs of disabled students, universities should ensure that the office bearers of HEPSN Centre include different kinds of disabled faculty members to represent and address the issues faced by various disabled students and faculty. Further, forming of student's committee to coordinate with other disabled students should also be made mandatory by universities, for more often than not there exists a huge communicational gap between students and HEPSN Unit. This committee should encompass student representatives of different types of disabled students so as to represent their distinct issues and needs.

Admission

Each admission process from advertising to placement of students shall be carried out only in consultation with the Central Committee for the Disabled, which shall also closely monitor the implementation of 5% reservation, equal distribution of seats among different category of disabled candidates, presence of sufficient information about facilities and provisions available for the disabled students in the advertisement brochure, publication of the admission brochure and application forms in accessible formats, and conduct of entrance test and interviews with scribes, sign language interpreters and other facilities.

The Central Committee shall also ensure using its own resources as well as those of other wings that special communication is rendered to the disabled applicants regarding the admission process and that adequate assistance is kept ready for the disabled candidates entering the university campus seeking admission. It shall also obtain a detailed report on the admission of disabled students in each department, centre and school of the university from the respective committees for the disabled, containing in addition an individualised assessment of each disabled student's requirements at the technical, physical, psychological and educational levels.

The committees in each department and school shall ensure that at least 5% of total seats are filled with disabled students with equal distribution among the different categories of disabled applicants. They shall assist each disabled student in filling up the required papers, payment of fees, contacting and finding admission to hostel and familiarising with the library, HEPSN Centre, Special Resource Centre and transport facilities. At least one member of the Central Committee shall be present during hostel admission to ensure no disabled student is denied residential accommodation and rooms are provided to the best convenience of the disabled students with accessible toilets and easy navigation with assistive devices like customised wheel chairs.

Teaching and Learning

Based on the recommendations of the Central Committee, the university administration shall issue circulars, orders and guidelines for making teaching and learning process disabled friendly in every sense. The Central Committee, on its own capacity, shall circulate detailed instructions and guidelines detailing out the ways in which teaching and learning could be optimised for each category of disabled students. Ramps, lifts, tactile footpath, braille signboards, audio-visual signals and specific such needs shall be made available for the disabled for accessing classrooms, labs, libraries and resource centres. The department level committees shall ask for the sign language interpreters, readers, special software applications and other special needs for their departments as and when required, and the Central Committee and HEPSN Resource Centre shall assist with the same in a timely manner. For this purpose, the Central Committee shall make sufficient availability of trained sign language interpreters, assistive software applications, recording devices, braille embossers and other facilities with funding from the university and other external sources. Digital screens, smart boards, audio descriptions, captions and other required assistive devices shall be used in classroom teaching, even if only a single disabled student is present in that class. The Central Committee shall ensure that the books are provided in most accessible formats to the disabled students from the library and HEPSN Resource Centre. The special trainers at the HEPSN Resource Centre shall orient the disabled students to learn using assistive technologies required for them to keep till they leave the campus.

Curriculum and Examination

The university administration, the Central Committee and the departmental committees shall ensure that no part of the curriculum is against the spirit and practice of inclusion of the disabled into mainstream society. They shall encourage programs, papers and courses of different kind for sensitising the nondisabled students about disability and disabled people's rights in a view to helping for their progress and overall growth. Examinations shall be conducted for the disabled students and Scribe facility for the blind shall be rendered as per the Guidelines for the Conduct of Written Examinations for Persons with Disabilities (Government of India, 2013), and committees of respective departments shall create a pool of scribe volunteers for this purpose. exemption from second language for the deaf, exemption from written exams and conduct of oral and convenient exam for intellectually disabled students can prove fruitful towards their inclusion.

Administration

The Central Committee can take up the responsibility of ensuring easy access of disabled students to all sections of the administrative unit of university. The persons in charge of each section and working staff should be intensively and convincingly trained so as to have a thorough knowledge about the rights and entitlements of disabled students, and the Central Committee can contribute by conducting periodic orientation programs/workshops towards this end. Making administrative communications and instructions available in accessible formats for each disabled student based on his/her convenience should be made an integral and inevitable part of the university functioning, again with contributions from the HEPSN unit. The Central Committee shall also ensure that university websites, circulars and documents remain accessible for all categories of disabled students.

Residence

The Central Committee can be consulted and its guidance shall be followed while building hostels and other places of residence inside the university. All hostels can be bestowed with provisions for lifts, ramps, tactile and sign indicators for navigating the building and other disabled friendly facilities as and when required. As the practice with a few Indian universities, certain number of rooms on the ground floor shall be kept reserved for disabled students in each hostel, and they shall first be filled with students having walking difficulties, followed by other disabled students if they opt for. Nondisabled hostel mates and disabled students shall be offered orientation and counselling by the HEPSN Unit for accommodating and socialising better with each other. Each hostel canteen shall have a staff and a group of student volunteers devoted to assist the disabled students while dining.

Campus Navigation and Access

Entire area of the campus, including each building and surrounding landscape, shall be made accessible for all kind of disabled students. International guidelines for universal design of buildings and transport facilities (United Nations, 2008) shall be strictly followed, of course with innovations for further enhancement and in order to fit the cultural and environmental contexts. The Central Committee shall be included as one of the key parts while planning and executing campus related activities such as building construction, transport arrangements, laying roads, setting up gardens, parks and play grounds, and conducting events. Technology can be put to best use for making campus navigation easier. In Pondicherry University, for instance, an android app *Vilosen* has been developed by a team of volunteers with guidance and support from the HEPSN Centre. This app informs the visually impaired where they stand inside the campus and lists out the nearby places with walking directions (Sivaraman, 2014). The same team has also developed an electronic device for the hearing impaired with which deaf students can get sign directions for reaching any building within the University campus. Even though these are experimental attempts with limited success, such initiatives can go a long way in transforming the way in which university campuses accommodate disabled students.

Students' Activities

Rather keeping the disabled students at the receiving end of all services, their representation in the students' union and participation in decision making shall be ensured by the Central Committee. Without patronising individual disabled students of course, the Committee shall make sure that at least one executive member of the student union will be disabled, and one seat each from all schools and departments is reserved for the disabled students, with proportional sharing among each kind of disability. (Such an arrangement is already in place at the English and Foreign Languages University) (Students' Union Election Commission, 2017). Thanks to vibrant disability activism, Jawaharlal Nehru University (JNU) has been successfully conducting online elections for the student body in accessible methods, and similar pattern can be adopted by all Indian universities. The students' union shall have regular meetings with the disabled students for understanding and representing their legitimate demands.

Placement Opportunities

The HEPSN Centre, in collaboration with university Placement Cell, shall ensure equal employment opportunities for disabled students. This can be effectively carried out by the Placement Officer appointed in the HEPSN Centre as per the UGC policy. The centre shall also strive to bring corporate companies, schools and human resource officers from other establishments to the campus so as to create employment opportunities. In addition to creating external contacts, the centre, with the financial assistance from universities, shall try to conduct sporadic coaching classes to clear state and central government exams.

CONCLUSION

By strengthening the HEPSN Centre with adequate funding, support and resources, by establishing a Central Committee and local level committees attached to the Central Committee for the disabled students, an accessible and resilient environment in the university can become a reality in India in near future. As an alternate to the present system of relegating every disability related issue to the HEPSN Centre (that has yielded only a little progress), we propose a model in which the committee can address the issues and needs of disabled students while their resource needs can be fulfilled by the HEPSN Centre.

Lack of awareness about disability, funding cuts, attitudinal barriers and patronizing attitudes among administrative authorities have marginalized the HEPSN Unit from the central functioning of universities. Only through centralizing the HEPSN Unit, can universities address the wide-spread issue of accessibility, attitudinal barriers and discriminations, for the Indian society is highly complex and stratified in terms of caste, class, religion, culture and language. Indian universities must find the ways and means of making their campuses barrier-free and productive places by focusing on equal opportunity, accessibility and consideration for intersectional categories of disabled students.

REFERENCES

Bansal, S. (2016, July 16). Census 2011 records rise in literacy among disabled. *The Hindu*. Retrieved from http://www.thehindu.com/news/national/Census-2011-records-rise-in-literacy-among-disabled/article14491381.ece

Chander, J. (2008). The role of residential schools in shaping the nature of the advocacy movement of the blind in India. In S. L. Gabel, & S. Danforth (Eds.), *Disability & the politics of education: An international reader* (pp. 201–224). New York, NY: Peter Lang.

Gabel, S. L., & Danforth, S. (Eds.). (2008). *Disability & the politics of education: An international reader.* New York, NY: Peter Lang.

Government of India. (2013). *Guidelines for conducting written examinations for persons with disabilities.* New Delhi: Ministry of Human Resource development.

Hindustan Times. (2017, November 16). With not even one per cent being disabled-friendly, colleges are difficult to access for many. *Editorial.* Retrieved from https://www.hindustantimes.com/editorials/with-not-even-one-per-cent-being-disabled-friendly-colleges-are-difficult-to-access-for-many/story-zfemcOhIWQhxiAVT1YNwWK.html

Jameel, S. S. (2011). Disability in the context of higher education: Issues and concerns in India. *Electronic Journal for Inclusive Education, 2*(7). Retrieved from https://corescholar.libraries.wright.edu/ejie/

Mehrotra, N. (2013). Disability, gender and caste intersections in Indian economy. In S. N. Barnartt, & B. M. Altman (Eds.), *Disability and intersecting statuses* (Research in Social Science and Disability, Vol. 7), (pp. 295–324). Bingley, UK: Emerald.

National Center for Education Statistics. (2016). *Digest of education statistics, 2015.* U.S. Department of Education. Retrieved from: https://nces.ed.gov/pubs2016/2016014.pdf

Saksena, S. & Sharma, R. (2015). Deconstructing barriers to access higher education: A cases study of students with disabilities in University of Delhi. *Journal of Undergraduate Research and Innovation, 1*(2), 316–337.

Shahi, A. (2016, April 26). Universities do little to enable the disabled. *Hindustan Times.* Retrieved from https://www.hindustantimes.com/analysis/universities-do-little-to-enable-the-disabled/story-0ivq04mDi5onH7pHF1JjWP.html

Sivaraman, R. (2014, December 18). An app that appropriately helps to navigate along campus. *The Hindu.* Retrieved from http://www.thehindu.com/todays-paper/tpnnational/tp-tamilnadu/an-app-that-appropriately-helps-to-navigate-along-campus/article6703161.ece

Students' Union Election Commission. (2017). *The English and foreign languages university students' union election notification 2017.* Hyderabad, India: English and Foreign Languages University.

Tilak, J. B. (2015). How inclusive is higher education in India? *Social Change, 45*(2), 185–223.

United Nations. (2008). Convention on the rights of persons with disabilities. Retrieved from https://www.un.org/development/desa/disabilities/convention-on-the-rights-of-persons-with-disabilities/convention-on-the-rights-of-persons-with-disabilities-2.html

University Grants Commission. (2008a). *Higher education in India: Issues related to expansion, inclusiveness, quality and finance.* New Delhi, India: University Grants Commission.

University Grants Commission. (2008b). https://www.yumpu.com/en/document/view/27292653/summary-of-ugc-xi-plan-guidelines-providing-financial-assistance-

PART III
GETTING ACCESS, ASSERTING RIGHTS

CHAPTER 17

If Not Now, When? Catalyzing Solidarity for Enduring Belonging in Higher Education

LAURA YVONNE BULK AND NEERA R. JAIN

INTRODUCTION

This is a moment for change. There have been many moments across history when the potential for change has been realized. Our moment of global crisis, fueled by the COVID-19 pandemic, has become one of those. Disabled people and those from other equity-deserving groups have been disproportionately affected by the effects of the global COVID-19 pandemic, and those embodying intersections of these positions experience the worst effects. Concurrently, pandemics of injustice, including racism, colonial legacies, and climate crises, have been highlighted. Having seen in real-time the devastating impact of injustice on a global scale, the need for transformative change is undeniable. Through this devastation it has been clear that Disabled people have something unique to offer, to guide us through uncertainty and illuminate alternate paths.

We have witnessed rapid change within universities in pandemic times from our vantage point in health professions education. The vitality of solidary, presence of interdependence, and benefits of flexibility have bubbled forth as major themes, in the interests of greater equity. Looking forward, we wonder, what changes will endure? Who will be centered as we move through and beyond this current crisis? And, how can we orient higher education towards a more just future?

This chapter celebrates some of the Disabled wisdom brought to the fore within higher education that warrants holding on to, while noting challenges that endure and deserve further attention. We explore ways to embrace this moment as catalysis to push us toward a future *with* Disability. In this future, different ways of knowing are embraced—Including experiential expertise, Indigenous knowledges, and other marginalized wisdoms. We argue that such a future requires stronger solidarities among equity-deserving groups to realize a university time and place when we are not just included, but we *belong with one another.*

This moment in history is globally unique across sectors, including in higher education. As higher education, in particular health professions education, is our sphere of influence, we will turn our attention there. In this chapter we set forth with open hands to share some of what we are learning, and to invite you into this journey of co-creating what the future will be and how solidarity, interdependence, and flexibility will inform a future that centers and celebrates what has been the margins.

TO LEARN AND TO CHANGE

Learning and change are relational processes, and as such we begin this chapter with an introduction of what brings each of the authors to the writing. As I (Neera) learn, I am constantly unlearning. I often feel caught between my values, ideals, and intellectual understandings and the automatic responses patterned through social learning and institutional structures. This ensnarement leaves me continually feeling never quite enough, and insufficient to the task. In this tension I can see most clearly the distance yet to travel to realize anti-ableism, decolonization, and other stances towards a more just world. To shift requires multi-layered work: internal examination and systemic disruption to pattern new ways of working into being. While much of my academic and professional focus has been systemic, lately, perhaps as a result of the pandemic, I find myself returning inward. Realizing anew how internalized colonial values of independence bred judgement and resistance to my family's culturally Indian ways of interdependence, blocking my ability to lean into living otherwise. Realizing, too, how I am still subservient to ableist systems in my design of classrooms and conferences, too easily letting go of my commitments in the face of institutional inertia. While I reckon internally with myself, I have found productive liberation in collectivity. Working together lightens the load; possibility becomes clearer and we hold each other accountable. Working deeply with others broadens collective expectations, as we build solidarity. I wish I did not need to be told, but I cherish those who call me in. Realizing interdependence, solidarity, and justice requires understanding that I am a work in (relational) progress, I (we) cannot succeed alone, we create a new world together.

Similarly, I (Laura) have felt, and often feel, inadequate to carry the weight of all I must learn, relearn, and unlearn if I want to be part of creating more just communities. Perhaps this sense that I will always have more space for growth in this area is as it should be. A femtor (a mentor working from female wisdom, knowledge base, and experience) (Brown, 2005; Lin, 2020) asked what my top values are, and humility was the first to come to mind. Humility to know that I will always have gaps in my learning and unlearning. To know that I *need* others. To know that *I* cannot find justice, justice is something *we* build together. Humility to serve others, to consider the needs and hopes of communities beyond my own as just as important as my own. Humility to realize that I only exist as a being in relationship and therefore I do not exist without you.

"Just show up." I was trying to understand how I could be in solidarity with Indigenous peoples, and this is the response an elder gave me. We need to show up for events, campaigns, parties, workshops, and so-on. Now a q-card with *"Show Up"* is fixed to my monitor as a frequent reminder that I need to be present and invite others to do the same. Sometimes that will mean spending spoons, taking time and physical and emotional energy. And that is when we have the chance to be gracious with one another, to be flexible, to embrace *crip time*, which centres the Disabled bodymind rather than the clock (Kafer, 2021), and to be part of decolonizing settler, neoliberal academia (Medak-Saltzman et al., 2022).

I am coming to understand that we need to belong with one another for our shared liberation and collective experience of justice. As we emerge into a new future, we need to create one in which the interdependence of lived experiences is part of our way of being in the world, and in which we embrace greater flexibility to adapt to the presence of more ways of knowing and being in the world. Our belonging, liberations, and very existence are bound up with one another and perhaps with the lands and waters in which we move. This interconnectedness led me to think about the vitality of solidarity.

FROM INTEREST CONVERGENCE TO SOLIDARITIES

> *"If you have come here to help me, you're wasting your time. If you have come because your liberation is bound up with mine, then let us work together." - Aboriginal activists group, Queensland, 1970s (Attributing Words, 2008)*

Throughout the height of the pandemic, individuals, groups, and institutions found themselves able to engage in ways they never expected. For example, we witnessed universities offer remote work integrated learning experiences to students across professions, and medical schools innovate new ways of engaging learners in virtual anatomy labs. These occurred because the "normies" have found themselves unable to engage in their *normal* ways of doing things, such learning through strictly in-person anatomy labs. The changes opened access for many Disabled people who were otherwise barred from certain experiences. For example, systemic inflexibility prevented students from engaging in anatomy labs when they were not well enough to attend in person and persistent physical inaccessibility limited some students access to fully engage in aspects of dissections.

While opening access is always a valuable end (Battalova et al., 2020; Iezzoni, 2016), the means to reaching that end varies. Interest convergence describes instances when access is opened because it serves the needs of the normies—a.k.a. (usually white, middle-class) non-disabled people (Annamma et al., 2013; Bell, 1980). This explains most of the access-enhancing changes that began at the outset of the pandemic. Those pushing for a *return to normal* in the wake of the (presumably "over") pandemic risk having these changes reversed and dismissed as unnecessary and untenable in the long-term. Interest convergence only works while the change continues to benefit the normies. Changes motivated solely by interest convergence are temporally fickle. An opportunity presented through the pandemic is to consider *going back to a new future*. This new future could include access-enhancing changes motivated by solidarities. Solidarity is a form of unity based on showing support for a shared interest or goal (*Solidarity*, 2022). In contrast to interest convergence, solidarities are about mutual benefit. Solidarities have the temporal longevity that interest convergence lacks. Through solidarities, we decenter the self and *my group*, instead turning our gaze to the wider community.

In the midst of global upheaval from 2020 through 2022, it became increasingly evident that an intersection lens is vital. For example, as groups declared that Black Lives Matter after police murdered George Floyd, those occupying the intersections interrogated: which Black lives? Disabled? (Kim, 2020) Trans? (Baloue, 2020). It also became clearer that solidarities are required for any of our lives to be bettered. We, as equity-deserving people, would not allow those silos to remain. We know that, as Erin Monahan said, "it is not our differences that separate us, but our reluctance to acknowledge them and to see the humanity still within our differences" (Monahan, 2021, para. 20). Through this time, (some) margins became centered, (some) ignored stories were told, (some) forgotten names were spoken. For example, some people with chronic physical health conditions had the opportunity to feel heard and perhaps somewhat understood when they talked about having to stay home to protect their health (Crystal, 2020). It became increasingly clear that "we can only truly understand ableism by tracing its connections to heteropatriarchy, white supremacy, colonialism, and capitalism" (Sins Invalid, 2020, para. 12).

As a social justice movement, we realize that we cannot stand, sit, roll, and walk apart, but must do so together. Our solidarities—being an ally or accomplice—must involve a commitment to listen, learn, act, and *show up*. Cross-movement solidarity is one of Disability Justice's ten key principles (Sins Invalid, 2019) and is closely connected with a view of the human subject as inherently interdependent. In this new future, access must be motivated by solidarity and predicated by the fact that we are interdependent beings. We can begin by building connections with other justice movements on campus, look for places where our interests align and where they diverge, show up to learn and support, and by amplifying others' interests alongside our own when getting the opportunity. For example, the Hybrid Access Now movement at the University of California Los Angeles, founded by students from the Disabled Student Union, the Mother Organizations Coalition, and Undergraduate Students Association Council at UCLA, together fought for more just conditions on intersectional, cross-movement grounds (Disabled Student Union UCLA & Mother Organizations of UCLA, 2022; UCLA Student Coalitions, 2022). This movement garnered support from across their campus and beyond that resulted in university-administration commitments to advance financial and structural support for BIPOC and disabled student interests, although not meeting all movement demands.

INTERDEPENDENCE

Within academia, neoliberal, ableist ideals hold sway over much of how things are done. Part of this ideal is the highly prized virtue of independence, defined as doing things alone and without assistance (Reindal, 1999, p. 353). Included in this concept of independence are the ways you teach, learn, research, and live. Researchers are expected to focus on their independent productivity to gain security in their academic jobs. Students are expected to know how to study from textbooks and perform independently on assessments of their knowledge, competence, and skill. Similarly, scholars are encouraged to present themselves as independent experts, who "know" alone rather than in community. This sets a false standard because the way independence is understood presumes that it means doing and being alone, which is untenable., From a Disabled perspective, learners, researchers, and scholars are already interdependent. Moreover, in contrast with a health professional's perspective, a cripped understanding of *independence* may be defined "as an ability to be in control of and make decisions about one's life" (Reindal, 1999, p. 353), which includes the notion of *interdependence.*

The experience of a global pandemic challenged the notion that individuals and their needs and desires are independent of one another. It became clear that our wellbeing may, in fact, be bound-up with that of others, including the environment. Climate change has foregrounded that the health of individuals and human communities is not independent of the health of non-human lands and animals. For example, movements against anti-Blackness have demanded that we realize we cannot claim that *all lives matter* until we reckon with the ways some are systematically devalued in our current societies. We must remedy the ways our societies and all lives within them suffer when we fail to protect certain lives.

The primacy of interdependence is prominent in Disability communities and in many Indigenous cultures. Thomas King explains that for Indigenous peoples across Turtle Island, the concept rendered in English as "all my relations" recognizes the interdependent web of kinship between peoples, animals, lands, and waters. It "is an encouragement for us to accept the responsibilities we have within the universal family by living our lives in a harmonious and moral manner." (King, 1990, p. ix) In te ao Māori (the world view of the Indigenous peoples of Aotearoa New Zealand) the value of *whanaungatanga* reflects an interdependent way of being and doing, defined as "relationship, kinship, sense of family connection—a relationship through shared experiences and working together which provides people with a sense of belonging" (Moorefield, 2022, n.p.). The Māori scholar Jacquie Kidd offers that connecting with people and understanding where they come from "is like breathing" (2015, p. 136). Against demands for independence that view interdepenent ways as weak and supplicating, Kidd explains, "whanaungatanga takes vulnerability and creates strength. It takes a single person and locates them/me within a vast network of bodies, histories, mythologies and vision. My weaknesses are known, but so are my strengths; both will energise, support, and inspire my life and work" (2015, p. 136).

Within Disability cultures, we know that "we need each other," (Mingus, 2010, para. 9) as the Disabled activist and thought leader Mia Mingus writes, "every time we turn away from each other, we turn away from ourselves" (2010, para. 9). Interdependence is one of the Disability Justice movement's ten key principles (Sins Invalid, 2019). Our liberation is bound up together. With the challenge lodged against the ideal of independence through the pandemic, movements for racial justice, and inequitably-distributed impacts of climate change, what can higher education learn from the wisdom of interdependence? What can interdependence do to shift how we think about educational spaces? What might centering this crip, Indigenous wisdom in higher education communities do? This might lead us to explore and re-examine: what and how we assess; conceptualizations of expertise, excellence, and competence; mutual care in classroom communities; and the ways we learn together—all as teachers and learners.

FLEXIBILITY

Our professional and lived experiences tell us that the rigidity of course, program, and degree design is a frequent challenge in higher education, in particular in professional degree programs with lock-step curricula. Courses may be tightly sequenced, available only at specific times, require in-person attendance, with assessment through specific means, all of which are framed by preset timescapes. These requirements demand learners conform to these expectations and presuppose certain bodyminds, finances, relational ties, and care duties (or lack thereof). That is, by requiring particular modes of becoming a professional, educational programs tend to privilege specific ways of knowing, being, and doing, and thereby prevent certain bodyminds from belonging.

The COVID-19 pandemic disrupted some of the rigid ways of "doing university education" previously treated as sacred. With in-person close contact deemed risky, most face-to-face instruction shifted to online and hybrid delivery. In health professions education, this opened the possibility for virtual clinical rotations, rounds, and educational events (Wallon et al., 2022). Activities like exams and medical residency interviews moved online, allowing for greater environmental control, cost and energy savings, and greater privacy (Hanes et al., 2022; Wallon et al., 2022). Timescapes were also revised in light of Zoom fatigue, heightened stress, distraction, and resource constraints caused by lockdowns and disease surges through practices such as blanket extensions and alternate course delivery. These practices transformed previously rigid environments and suggest the possibility for *flexibility*, offering varied ways to engage with university education.

Flexibility is a key tenet of universal design approaches, wherein environments are designed for maximum inclusivity. A strategy that emerged from Disabled activist movements for disability-led design of material objects and physical spaces (Hamraie, 2016), universal design has since been applied broadly, for example, event and learning-environment design. The Universal Design for Learning (UDL) framework, for example, centers flexibility in its call for multiple means of action, expression, and representation in learning spaces (CAST, 2018). The approach builds in alternatives, assuming learners with varied capacities and preferences. Universal design approaches contrast with dominant paradigms of university access driven by retrofitting individualized accommodations. Frustratingly revelatory, many of the rapid shifts during the pandemic reflected changes Disabled people were previously told were impossible (A., 2020; Hamraie, 2020). Prior to the pandemic, such changes were evaluated as individual requests deemed to "fundamentally alter" course requirements. For example, we are aware of a chronically-ill student who required a remote clinical placement and was told in early March 2020 that this accommodation was impossible. In mid-March 2020 that non-option suddenly became the only option for all students. Reflecting interest convergence, these (im)possibilities only became everyday practices when they benefitted those deemed the majority.

ONGOING CHALLENGES

Despite the potential benefits of greater flexibility revealed through the COVID-19 pandemic, challenges have endured. Pandemic flexibility did not always recognize co-existing inequities, such as access to high-quality internet, assistive technology, and quiet space, as well as care responsibilities. Alternate delivery did not necessarily correct pre-existing lacuna in access thinking, for example, assuming visual capability during online course delivery via screen-share rather than describing images or reading aloud critical text (Hanes et al., 2022). Newly flexible learning environments represented *crisis design*, rapid shifts in pedagogy made due to urgent collective necessity with minimal training, time, and infrastructure, under stressful conditions (Hodges et al., 2020). The quality and sustainability of flexible education delivered was, at times, questionable and failed to level the playing field.

The pandemic is demonstrating that increased flexibility is possible, and we argue it ought to be retained into the future. Such flexibility benefits not just Disabled people, but also those with work, care, and community responsibilities, while supporting ongoing public health efforts (e.g., not coming to class when sick). Some changes may be easily retained, while others require additional resources. Institutional funding for tools to facilitate genuine, high-quality flexibility is needed. For example, infrastructure to facilitate hybrid learning, such as classroom cameras and area microphones, would facilitate more fluid interactions between learners in and out of the he creation of time and space to build educator skills in flexibility by design would recognize that this approach requires a mindful shift that necessitates new tools. Institutions, programs, faculty, and campus services must review and revise policies to incorporate flexibility, ensuring that rigidity is rooted out of structures. Institutional investment and community partnerships are needed to assist students who need technology (e.g., strong internet connection) to effectively engage in hybrid learning, thus facilitating equitable access for all students to the benefits of the movement towards flexibility.

CONCLUSION

The higher education community needs to engage in a more fundamental, critical exploration of the goals of education to avoid a patchwork approach that simply appends access or anti-racism work. We must consider how current configurations reflect ableist, racist, cis/hetero/patriarchal, and colonial assumptions that require transformation. Flexibility aligned with a universal design approach that advocates broad, intersectional accessibility could activate anti-racist and anti-ableist values when led by lived insights of those most marginalized by current systems (Dolmage, 2017; Hamraie, 2013, 2016; Waitoller & King Thorius, 2016). Access must also be dynamic, embodying Dolmage's (2017) assertion that universal design is a verb, an ongoing and deeply relational process—not a point on the horizon achieved through checklists or singular gestures. While accommodations are likely always necessary to ensure access, prioritizing universal design would help to address intersectional inequities activated by current accommodation-focused approaches (A., 2020; Krebs, 2019). An interdependent, solidarity-driven, and active approach to education could also forge more connected community through the recognition that we are stronger, learn more, and learn better when we do so together.

As you reflect on this chapter, we invite you to consider your practice and expectations in relation to the following questions:

- What new educational design elements, such as flexibility, were introduced during the COVID-19 pandemic? How and where might greater flexibility support your participation in higher education spaces? How can we meaningfully and sustainably retain flexibility going forward to support your ongoing participation?
- In what ways are our classes, programs, policies, and structures rigid, allowing limited ways to engage in education? How might we introduce choice and control into these elements, for everyone?
- What do equity-deserving groups articulate as current barriers and how are they currently working around them? What would work better?
- How do you engage in cross-movement solidarity?
- In what ways do you 'show up'?

We acknowledge that many in our higher education communities are exhausted by the (currently ongoing) pandemic. We embrace the emotions that come with this. We witness the statements of people who feel they have no time or energy left to work toward *ideals* of justice, equity, diversity, and inclusion principles. However, we argue that these are not ideals, but imperatives. In this time, it has become clear that moving forward as a world requires us to build societies and institutions that dismantle oppressions and act toward more just relationships. Arguably, there has never been a better time for massive change. If not now, when? We are primed, it is time!

REFERENCES

A., R. (2020). *The burden and consequences of self-advocacy for disabled BIPOC*. Disability Visibility Project. https://disabilityvisibilityproject.com/2020/07/19/the-burden-and-consequences-of-self-advocacy-for-disabled-bipoc/

Annamma, S. A., Connor, D., & Ferri, B. (2013). Dis/ability critical race studies (DisCrit): theorizing at the intersections of race and dis/ability. *Race Ethnicity and Education*, *16*(1), 1–31. https://doi.org/10.1080/13613324.2012.730511

Attributing Words. (2008). Unnecessary evils. http://unnecessaryevils.blogspot.com/2008/11/attributing-words.html

Baloue, S. (2020). *On transgender day of remembrance, remember that black trans lives matter, too*. https://www.them.us/story/transgender-day-of-remembrance-black-trans-lives-matter-tony-mcdade-layleen-cubilette-polanco

Battalova, A., Bulk, L. Y., Nimmon, L., Hole, R., Krupa, T., Lee, M., Mayer, Y., Jarus, T., Hole, R., Krupa, T., Lee, M., & Jarus, T. (2020). "I can understand where they're coming from": How clinicians' disability experiences shape their interaction with clients. *Qualitative Health Research*, *30*(13), 2064–2076. https://doi.org/10.1177/1049732320922193

Bell, D. A. (1980). Brown v. Board of education and the interest-convergence dilemma. *Harvard Law Review*, *93*(3), 518. https://doi.org/10.2307/1340546

Brown, R. N. (2005). *Between empowerment and marginalization*. University of Michigan.

CAST. (2018). *Universal design for learning guidelines version 2.2*. http://udlguidelines.cast.org

Crystal, J. (2020). *Learning to live well with a persistent illness*. Harvard Health Blog.

Disabled Student Union UCLA, & Mother Organizations of UCLA. (2022). *Longest sit-in in UCLA history ends with massive victory for students*. https://knock-la.com/ucla-disabled-students-union-sit-in/

Dolmage, J. T. (2017). *Academic ableism: Disability and higher education*. University of Michigan Press.

Hamraie, A. (2013). Designing collective access: A feminist disability theory of universal design. *Disability Studies Quarterly*, *33*(4).

Hamraie, A. (2016). Universal design and the problem of "Post-Disability" ideology. *Design and Culture*, *8*(3), 285–309. https://doi.org/10.1080/17547075.2016.1218714

Hamraie, A. (2020). *Accessible teaching in the time of COVID-19*. Critical Design Lab. https://www.mapping-access.com/blog-1/2020/3/10/accessible-teaching-in-the-time-of-covid-19

Hanes, J. E., Waserman, J. L., & Clarke, Q. K. (2022). The accessibility of virtual residency interviews: the good, the bad, the solutions. *Canadian Medical Education Journal*, *13*(2), 98–100. https://doi.org/10.36834/cmej.74107

Hodges, C., Moore, S., Lockee, B., Trust, T., & Bond, A. (2020). The difference between emergency remote teaching and online learning. *Educause Review*.

Iezzoni, L. I. (2016). Why increasing numbers of physicians with disability could improve care for clients with disability. *AMA Journal of Ethics*, *18*, 1041–1049.

Kafer, A. (2021). After crip, crip afters. *South Atlantic Quarterly*, *120*(2), 415–434. https://doi.org/10.1215/00382876-8916158

Kidd, J. (2015). Whanaungatanga is not an option: An autoethnography in two voices. In R. E. Rinehart, E. Emerald, & R. Matamua (Eds.), *Ethnographies in pan pacific research* (pp. 135–141). Routledge. https://doi.org/10.4324/9781315718927

Kim, S. (2020, July 3). Black disabled lives matter: We can't erase disability in #BLM. Teen Vogue. Retrieved from https://www.teenvogue.com/story/black-disabled-lives-matter.

King, T. (1990). *All my relations: An anthology of contemporary Canadian native fiction*. McClelland & Stewart Inc.

Krebs, E. (2019). Baccalaureates or burdens? Complicating 'Reasonable Accommodations' for American college students with disabilities. *Disability Studies Quarterly*, *39*(3). https://doi.org/10.18061/dsq.v39i3.6557

Lin, D. (2020). In search of a femtor: The complexities of female mentorship in academic medicine. *Southern Medical Journal*, *113*(10), 495–497. https://doi.org/10.14423/SMJ.0000000000001154

Medak-Saltzman, D., Misri, D., & Weber, B. (2022). Decolonizing time, knowledge, and disability on the tenure clock. *Feminist Formations*, *34*(1), 1–24. https://doi.org/10.1353/ff.2022.0000

Mingus, M. (2010). *Interdependence (excerpts from several talks)*. Leaving Evidence. https://leavingevidence.wordpress.com/2010/01/22/interdependency-exerpts-from-several-talks/

Monahan, E. (2021). *White-washed history, radical listening, and turning dialogue into action*. Terra Incognita. https://www.terraincognitamedia.com/features/white-washed-history-radical-listening-and-turning-dialogue-into-action2017

Moorefield, J. C. (2022). Whanaungatanga. In *Te aka Māori dictionary*.

Reindal, S. M. (1999). Independence, dependence, interdependence: Some reflections on the subject and personal autonomy. *Disability & Society*, *14*(3), 353–367. https://doi.org/10.1080/09687599926190

Sins Invalid. (2019). *Sin, tooth, and bone: The basis of our movement is people* (2nd ed.). Sins Invalid.

Sins Invalid. (2020). *What is disability justice?* Sins Invalid. https://www.sinsinvalid.org/news-1/2020/6/16/what-is-disability-justice

Solidarity. (2022). Merriam-Webster Dictionary. https://www.merriam-webster.com/dictionary/solidarity

UCLA Student Coalitions. (2022). *Hybrid access now: Statement by UCLA Student Coalitions*. Disability Visibility Project. https://disabilityvisibilityproject.com/2022/02/06/hybrid-access-now-statement-by-ucla-student-coalitions/

Waitoller, F. R., & King Thorius, K. A. (2016). Cross-pollinating culturally sustaining pedagogy and universal design for learning: Toward an inclusive pedagogy that accounts for dis/ability. *Harvard Educational Review*, *86*(3), 366–389.

Wallon, R. C., Gossett, J., & Meeks, L. M. (2022). It took a pandemic: Enduring lessons for improving accessibility in medical education. *Disability Compliance in Higher Education*, *27*(11), 1–15.

CHAPTER 18

Disabled by Society: Knowing and Invoking Your Rights

KATELIN ANDERSON AND BETH ROGERS

INTRODUCTION

Adaptations and accommodations are reasonable expectations for anyone, but it's easy for disabled people and graduate students to subconsciously feel like they're asking for a favour when making such a request. There's a harmful belief in many institutions that higher study should be exhausting and unforgiving, and that if a student needs accommodations to keep up with a gruelling set of demands (often demands that do nothing to add intellectual rigor or promote comprehensive learning), they don't belong in academia. Accommodations are often framed as leniency or unfair advantage, which ignores the reality that a lot of academia is constructed inaccessibly—even to many non-disabled people.

Students can break that falsehood by claiming the rights they already have to participate in an academic environment. All students deserve, and should be legally provided, equal opportunities not just to *be* a student, but to make the most of their time in studies—including graduate studies. In many places, to some extent, the right to not be discriminated against is enshrined in law. Previous efforts of students and other disabled activists have generated precedents to facilitate access. Knowing the laws that exist and the associated rights is essential to protecting them. As these laws will vary by place, this chapter offers a generalized overview that will be applicable to a wider audience: it will be up to the student to apply the advice to their culture/place of residence.

This chapter outlines legal rights and strategies for addressing conflicts of inaccessibility, written both for students and for university staff. There are two sets of guidelines that every student should know how to navigate: institutional and governmental. Institutional guidelines are set out by universities and apply only to that university, while governmental laws (whether federal or specific to state or province) tend to be broader and explicitly outline the rights of individuals. While the institutional guidelines will be of primary concern to individuals, in case of escalation, obfuscation, or injustice on the part of a university, it is good to have a passing familiarity with governmental laws.

It is not necessary to memorize every legislated right, but developing the skills of knowing how to locate, navigate, and invoke these rights and guidelines will make it easier to put together a clear, well-articulated case for access or resolving an unsatisfactory situation. If rights are not legally protected in a specific region, these skills will help find precedents that may still help, or to coordinate with people already working to protect these rights in that area.

In the section below, two anecdotes will illustrate how difficult these problems can be without support, before moving into strategies for addressing such issues. The names used for the students on which these anecdotes are based are pseudonyms. The experiences of "Rosalie" and "Annie," while based on actual people, are included to provide insight into the complicated, often understated nature of accessibility concerns in higher education. They additionally highlight the imperative to know and to freely access rights, the subject of the remainder of the chapter.

ROSALIE AND ANNIE

Rosalie, an autistic PhD candidate at a European university with a number of mood disorders, including depression and anxiety, was applying for government assistance to help with living expenses while continuing her studies. Her doctors advised her to leave her program in order to qualify, to prove that she was not capable of working. Up until that point, Rosalie had been able to work full-time as a student, which to her doctors and her institution meant that she did not really need accommodations. Besides the medical concerns, the ability to do scholarly work was a vital part of Rosalie's quality of life.

"At that time, they were not considering that what I study in school is a main interest of mine and is very tailored to my autistic needs and strengths," Rosalie said, "whereas any other job or even studying a different subject would be overwhelming for me and impossible. However, they did tell me that if I would just drop out of school then they would help me. [But] dropping out of school is the very last thing I wanted to do! It's one of the few things that bring me joy and without it I would be miserable. Even if dropping a semester might mean I could get my evaluation and get financial support, it would be dangerous to my depression and possibly my life."

Similarly, Annie faced a difficult personal choice that illustrates how lack of easy access to appropriate accommodations can make pursuing graduate education feel impossible. Annie planned to matriculate into a PhD program, but the deadline for her MA thesis at a European university loomed, and she already had several extensions. She hesitated to ask for more time, even though her pain was getting worse. Her headache disorder made it difficult to focus for long periods of reading, and screen brightness caused shooting pains. She could either request another extension and try to polish her thesis through more months of unabated pain and stress or she could finish the MA without the grade necessary to continue to a PhD.

Up until that point, things had been going well. Before starting the thesis portion of her program, she said, "I always got help to postpone my exams when needed. My teachers were understanding. But I always had to explain that I really wanted to learn as much as I could and do my best. I think that some of them thought that I was just lazy when they first met me because my disability isn't visible."

Annie felt she had to complete her MA thesis unsatisfactorily for the sake of her health. Efficiently completing her thesis was too hard to do without assistance or accommodations, like audio recordings of books, voice transcription software, or even an assistant, that might have helped. Merely having more time wasn't sufficient for her needs. The experience of being judged upon first meeting or having unreasonable demands placed upon them in the guise of helpful assistance is common for all who have disabilities. These assumptions can "lead to acts of commission or omission on the part of others that impose limits on the social participation of stigmatized individuals," which can further compound when imbalances of power are involved (Green et al., 2005, pp. 205–210). It goes hand-in-hand with the idea that it is incumbent on the disabled person to shoulder past difficulty through personal effort alone, telling them to either create their own accommodations or else eschew them entirely.

There are many examples of the ways that administrators and university staff may casually and unthinkingly undermine a disabled student's efforts to complete a degree (Titchkosky, 2008). These can range from the well-meaning, as in, "We put up accessibility signs and got a wheelchair ramp for the entrance!" (while bathrooms are still inaccessible) to the more upsetting, "If they can't use the bathrooms, *what are they doing here anyway?*" (Titchkosky, 2008, pp. 42–43).

What do students do when their disability becomes overwhelming and they question whether or not to continue? What can they do if, in extreme cases, someone denies them opportunities (or tries to) because of their disabilities? How do administrators or staff, who may or may not be disabled themselves, create a more adaptive environment?

LOCATING YOUR RIGHTS

The first step to take is to figure out what protections and rights disabled students have. It's important to find both institutional rules and governmental laws that may apply. Whether you're a student yourself, trying to find out what recourse you have in an already unfavorable situation, or a university staff member trying to establish fair policies ahead of time, this is a good place to start.

A quick internet search for "disability + [university name]" or "disability protections [country/region]" is probably the quickest way to locate documents pertaining to rights, and has the handy feature of allowing you to bookmark, print, or download regulations so that you can quickly reference them if necessary. Otherwise, call or visit your local government office (or disability-specific organization) and ask if they can provide you with a reference, or help you find the sections of law relevant to your needs. Don't be afraid to ask if they have a plain language version available, or if there's an expert who can help you with questions you might have.

It's increasingly common for universities to have some sort of disability services or assistance department. Even if you aren't sure you'll need their assistance, it is a good idea to make yourself familiar with this office, especially prior to the start of the academic period in case accommodations are needed (Rose, 2010). There's no guarantee that these people will be sympathetic to your particular situation, but their primary goal should be ensuring that all disabled people's rights are enforced. They may be able to offer you resources outlining your rights as a student or explain how the university deals with disability related situations. A good disability services office will also be able to explain how to make sure you and your needs are protected, whether any documentation is required, or what sorts of accommodations can be provided through the university. This is where Annie could have gone to ask what other accommodations she could have accessed, other than simply extended time for her thesis. Rosalie, likewise, could have asked this office for documentation of the accommodations she did have, or possibly spoken to someone about how other students in her position were able to secure the financial support they needed.

Some universities might ask for a doctor's sanction or documentation of a diagnosis for specific accommodations. If you don't have these things, or getting a diagnosis requires money that you don't have, ask if they have a process in place to assist with obtaining that documentation. There may be a fund students can apply to specifically in the service of seeing a doctor for a diagnosis for disability documentation. Even if you feel your disability is too minor to require much in the way of accommodations, if you're established with the disability services office, it will be that much easier to invoke your rights as a disabled student when you do need accommodations or run into problems. If your institution doesn't have such an office, consider contacting the Human Resources or equivalent personnel department for further resources.

Being aware of the rights of disabled people is beneficial to the institution, too. Beyond gaining a reputation as a fair and even-handed place of learning, there are pragmatic aspects for universities pre-emptively considering these issues. Ease of resolution is probably the major incentive to consider institutional policies and know the legal protections disabled people have in your region. Consulting the applicable federal agency for compliance or guidance beforehand can save you and the university support office time, money, and legal trouble in the long term when confronted with these issues.

Even if an institution has only recently established such an office, disability services professionals can look to resources and established groups for guidance. These resources include the international Association on Higher Education and Disability (AHEAD), and more localized organizations such as the Australian Disability Clearing House on Education and Training (ADCET), the Canadian Association of Disability Service Providers in Post-secondary Education (CADSPPE), or the European Disability Forum (EDF) (Oslund, 2015, pp. 56–58). There are likely other region-specific organizations, but disability services providers may find these collected resources helpful even in their own regions.

Institutions should have clear and accessible guidelines on what protections and rights disabled students and staff have. Issues of accommodation, especially in graduate work, can be a careful balance of meeting student rights of access and maintaining fair standards for graduate study across a number of different programs. If individual graduate programs have "essential requirements," or if an institution has overarching requirements for graduate study, a clear and available statement of these requirements would provide a structure for implementing accommodations and maintaining the academic rigor and integrity of graduate work (Rose, 2010). Ideally, the student should not have to search far to learn about their rights (or specific expectations of the graduate program). Universities should also outline their processes for requesting accommodations and dealing with rights violations. This provides disabled students and staff with an unambiguous course of redress and makes it simpler to resolve problems or to identify areas of policy that have been unintentionally unclear, open to misinterpretation, or are in conflict with federal law.

While having a clear website link or printed copies available in applicable offices are a good start, a simple language guide to these policies emailed out to all staff and students at the start of term or placed in orientation folders would be an easy and effective way to disseminate information. Plain language documents help provide clarity for everyone involved and help university staff apply policy consistently and effectively.

Ideally, the university will have a policy for addressing grievances, but if they haven't instituted one, there are some basic guidelines that the student can follow in order to invoke their rights and resolve any situation as best as possible. The exact implementation of the suggestions below will need to be interpreted to work in each academic culture.

INVOKING YOUR RIGHTS

Document everything. The moment you are denied access to a resource or opportunity, or something makes you uneasy, take notes. This documentation can be relatively informal in nature, but note the date, time, place, people involved, and substance of the issue as comprehensively as possible. Avoid jargon and field-specific terms for easy understanding, be as specific as possible, avoid speculation, and describe the effects of the behavior, whether that is describing a direct barrier to your academic progress or its emotional effect on you (Mitchell & Gamlem, 2017). Be sure to keep a backup of your documentation in secure location.

Do this in whatever manner is going to be most complete for you—some options are to hand write the notes as an incident report, to send an email to your professor (or colleague) recapping the meeting, or to vocally record as much as you can recall. It is inadvisable to record the conversation itself, as the legalities of doing so will vary by area. Unfortunately, most guidelines on such conflict documentation are geared toward Human Resource professionals, but looking up local HR handbooks may give you some insight into the regional standards and expectations for documentation. Consistent documentation makes these issues easier to resolve if they escalate, and prevents the conflict from turning into a vague "they said, I said" situation. If Annie were to have investigated additional accommodations, it likely would have been helpful to have any discussion about her extensions documented, to demonstrate what she'd already tried and why the extension alone hadn't been sufficient. She would seem organized and responsible, and would be able to show that there was a reasonable need that was insufficiently addressed.

Clarify the situation. The follow-up email or meeting is particularly helpful for this. When addressing the issue, ask specifically *why* they believe you can't participate or contribute: make them define the barriers to entry. Ask them to help you come up with adaptations that would circumvent these barriers, or begin to brainstorm accessible solutions yourself. Often, these denials are unfounded or based in unthinking assumptions about your capabilities. Asking the person you're working with to explain what they're thinking may be enough for them to reconsider their assumptions. If Rosalie had been able to get a clear answer as to why her studies supposedly proved she didn't need assistance, she would have been able to press a specific point, or ask about equivalent circumstances; that wouldn't have been a guarantee, but Rosalie would have had a definitive set of disqualifications to argue against, rather than a generalized denial.

Determine actionability. If the issue cannot be resolved independently, then discover whether the issue is actionable or which policies it might contradict. What jurisdiction does the grievance fall under? What recourse might you have to address it? Define your goals. Do you want access to a specific activity/resource or the skill/lesson/experience it would offer? Would you be willing to consider an alternative that provides you with the same end product? What, if anything, do you want to be done about the person or situation that incited your action? If you can clearly answer these questions, it may be easier to reach a resolution, and will help you explain why you're pursuing this matter. For example, if Annie could have clearly articulated the problems caused by her headache disorder and asked for specific accommodations (voice recognition software or print materials), she may have had more support, compared to just having more time. A disability services professional working with her could have used these same questions to help her describe where she was struggling, and suggested more apt aid.

Deescalate the situation. Generally, you want to diminish hostile feelings and keep matters from requiring official legal or institutional action. Approach with a mindset of giving the other party the benefit of the doubt. Creating rapport through positivity, receptive and engaged attitude, and remembering/underscoring mutual goals will foster better communications and outcomes, especially in face-to-face discussions (Nadler, 2003). As a disabled student or staff member, doing this will let you come across as reasonable, and assuming that someone involved wants to assist you will get you farther. This is especially true if the person who created the conflict is unapologetic or recalcitrant. If you still don't gain any traction, there's nothing wrong with explaining your frustration or going higher up: make use of the previous two steps heavily here. For Rosalie, the difficulty was feeling like she was getting nowhere, and it may have been worthwhile to appeal to higher authorities or to ask for help from those more familiar with her circumstances. For Annie, feeling like she needed to power through on her own as much as possible meant she was unable to get the help to achieve her goals, when she had legitimate reasons to ask for something more. Deescalation is about reducing interpersonal friction, not about conceding your rights.

The institution involved in a grievance should know that a potentially protracted dispute can be more easily resolved by assuming that the student has reasonable requests and wants to work with you. If a student has trouble articulating the problem, refer them to the questions in the previous two sections. An institution's policy should try to deescalate a situation, but if it isn't going to work, there needs to be a clear process on how to proceed without prioritizing institutional pride over the educational needs of the disabled student.

Pursue equitable solutions. This point is more relevant to institutions, but is an important consideration for everyone involved in these conversations. Recall that almost anything can be adapted for various needs, whether those are specific, tangible classroom resources or more abstract experiences. Be open to discussion from students pursuing accommodation or redress as suggested above—there may be less obvious accommodation options that maintain academic rigor while also meeting the needs of the student. As someone working at an institution, whether in administration or as an instructor, consider making it part of the guidelines that staff need to consider or even pre-emptively take this step. Annie's case is a good example of this: an instructor who was more familiar with these issues might have been able to address the underlying concerns when Annie initially brought up the need for an extension.

Encouraging staff to plan adaptations for various accessibility issues—or doing such an exercise yourself—can increase flexible thinking that's more inclusive of disabled students. While universal design for learning/instruction (UDL/UDI) principles have largely been explored in undergraduate studies, the focus on flexibility and emphasis on anticipating the need for "alternatives, options, and adaptations to meet the challenge of diversity" would provide structure for educators and institutions wanting to implement these principles in graduate education, benefitting not only disabled graduate students, but also their nondisabled peers (Rose et al., 2006, p. 2). Institutional training opportunities in disability awareness and support is a key factor in faculty attitude toward implementing these principles (Lombardi et al., 2013), and may decrease resistance to being asked to accommodate or adapt in the future, potentially averting future conflicts.

Even with these efforts, non-disabled (or differently disabled) administrators or professors may not always propose equitable or fully considered solutions to the student's concerns. You may be offered a solution that doesn't resolve the situation or seems insulting or counterproductive even so. Rosalie's problem is certainly one of these, but she still has the option of reaching out to disability organizations like those mentioned at the beginning of the chapter. While you might be (understandably) frustrated, try not to escalate the situation immediately. Sometimes, it can be as simple as pointing out to an advisor/trusted mentor that an offered alternative or suggestion sets a bad precedent, has unfair implications, or defeats the purpose of the goal. Try to redirect focus to making sure you are able to attain that goal, rather than on the administration being discriminatory to greater or lesser degrees, however true that may be. Asking for a fair solution to a problem, not just *any* solution to a problem, is not unreasonable.

CONCLUDING THOUGHTS

Not everything can clearly be discussed in terms of rights and discrimination, and sometimes genuinely harmful actions or beliefs may not be considered legally actionable. That doesn't mean that the problems themselves can't be navigated. Take the time to consider how you are going to manage the specific difficulties you might encounter as a disabled graduate student.

What happens, for example, when a professor believes that someone cannot or—or should not—pursue a PhD because of their disability? "I don't think you'd make a good PhD student because you're disabled and it would be too hard for you, so I won't write you a recommendation" is a lot harder to fight institutionally than, "If you can't get into the lecture theater, you're just going to have to miss that seminar and lose credit." Or, like Rosalie, you may find that succeeding academically means people perceive you as not being "truly disabled." For higher-level biases and predicaments, many of strategies above still apply, though they may be more draining when you don't have a clear guideline or policy to point to.

Institutions need to actively work against apathy and assumptions. Don't just have guidelines, but listen to faculty and students who are disabled to find the flaws in the current system. Create a university culture that actively strives to be adaptable in design, rather than retrofitting accommodations at the last minute. Strive not just to match the letter but the spirit of the law when it comes to disability protections.

Navigating these biases from either side is exhausting, draining work. Whether you're dealing with a personal struggle or are coping with difficult doctors or university staff, cultivate your support network, even within your university. You'd be hard pressed to find disabled members of academia who *haven't* struggled with these conflicts, and the rights that you can invoke were enshrined by the hard work of disabled people and their allies who came before you.

When you know your rights and know how to navigate them, when you assume that you have earned your space in academia and have the right to adaptations that allow you to access that space, when you have the tools to negotiate challenges to that right of access, you take the burden off your future-self so that they can deal with the conflict in front of them with surety.

REFERENCES

Green, S., Davis, C., Karshmer, E., Marsh, P., & Straight, B. (2005). Living stigma: The impact of labeling, stereotyping, separation, status loss, and discrimination in the lives of individuals with disabilities and their families. *Sociological Inquiry, 75*(2), 197–215.

Lombardi, A., Murray, C., & Dallas, B. (2013). University faculty attitudes toward disability and inclusive instruction: Comparing two institutions. *Journal of Postsecondary Education and Disability, 26*(3), 221–232.

Mitchell, B., & Gamlem, C. (2017). *The big book of HR*. Wayne, NJ: Career Press.

Nadler, J. (2003). Rapport in negotiation and conflict resolution. *Marquette Law Revue, 87*(4), 875–882.

Oslund, C. M. (2015). *Disability services and disability studies in higher education: History, contexts, and social impacts*. New York, NY: Palgrave MacMillan.

Rose, D. H., Harbour, W. S., Johnston, C. S., Daley, S. G., & Abarbanell, L. (2006). Universal design for learning in postsecondary education: Reflections on principles and their application. *Journal of Postsecondary Education and Disability, 19*(2), 135–151.

Rose, M. (2010). Accommodating graduate students with disabilities (Working Paper No. 830). Retrieved from http://cou.on.ca/papers/accommodating-graduate-students-with-disabilities/

Titchkosky, T. (2008). "'To pee or not to pee?'" Ordinary talk about extraordinary exclusions in a university environment. *The Canadian Journal of Sociology/Cahiers Canadiens de Sociologie, 33*(1), 37–60.

CHAPTER 19

Identifying and Eliminating Digital Barriers after COVID

KAREN McCALL

INTRODUCTION

"After COVID, it's much harder for us to hold to the comforting illusion that ableism is mostly unintentional and benign." (Pulrang, 2021) By the time the COVID-19 pandemic was waning in 2022, there were no more unintentional digital barriers. The experience of a global pandemic in a digital age resulted in exposing the depth and breadth of the intentional barriers created as we, the global community, invented and advanced technology. as we advanced technology, we lost the sense of inclusion that was an integral part of inventions before the advent of computer technology.

Components of our daily interactions with digital technology have their roots in inclusive inventions. For example, the typewriter was invented in Italy by someone who wanted to help his friend who was blind communicate with family and friends. In the patent application for the phonograph, Thomas Edison stated that the phonograph would be helpful for people who are blind because books could be placed on the cylinders and read aloud. The telephone, invented by Alexander Graham Bell was an assistive technology to help his wife, who was hard of hearing, communicate with her family and friends. Even e-mail which is both an essential component and the bane of our existence was further developed by a scientist using e-mail before the broader use of the Internet for public consumption, as an assistive technology for his wife who was deaf as a way of communications. Yet, as the Internet and its Internet of Things evolved, people with disabilities have been intentionally left behind.

We've known since at least 1998–1999 when the first Web Content Accessibility Guidelines (WCAG 1.0) were published by the World Wide Web consortium, that people with disabilities were being left behind. Section 508 in the United States (2002) legislated web accessibility but left out digital accessibility as an encompassing concept.

There is a common misperception that if something is in print, or if it is on a computer screen, then it is accessible. Theoretically, the only barriers that should exist are those related to the physical environment. However, digital environments or content are not currently inherently accessible to people who are blind or who have visual, learning, cognitive, information processing, or print disabilities. An analogy can be made to building a house. If the house doesn't use universal design principles incorporated into building codes and legislation, that minimize any further renovations to make the house accessible for people with disabilities, it has been built to exclude people with disabilities.

When the first wave of COVID-19 spanned the globe in January 2020, the shift in recognition of the level of exclusion was immediate and devastating for most faculty and students with disabilities (Anderson, 2020). While higher education campuses provided access to high-speed Internet, alternate text production services, libraries, and other student support services; once back in their hometowns or isolated in place outside of the campus bubble, students encountered chaos and insurmountable barriers to education.

This chapter provides insights into intentional digital barriers faced by students, faculty, and staff who are blind, visually disabled, or who have a learning, cognitive, information processing, or print disability. Readers will walk away with a clearer understanding of how a global pandemic revealed a "Grand Canyon" sized digital divide in accessing higher education. It remains to be seen whether there is enough synergy to lessen the divide or eliminate it.

Readers will be more equipped to ask for, or demand, appropriate software and accessible document design training at their institutions. It is hoped that faculty who have experienced digital barriers first-hand encountered when the educational landscape shifted to an online-only model of delivery that removes any comfort level within 24 to 48 hours, will retain those experiences, and engage in self-learning and advocacy toward inclusive education.

Finally, this chapter offers clear suggestions on how institutions can, and must, take a leadership role in eliminating those barriers.

ACCESS TO THE INTERNET AND BROADBAND

With the advent of the COVID-19 pandemic, the gulf between those who had access to high-speed Internet and those who did not was spread over a broader range of populations. Living in south-western Ontario Canada, it wasn't unusual to hear that one side of a street had high-speed Internet while the other side of the street did not. Access to the Internet was not dependent on affluence or social position, but literally on which side of the street you lived on. Internet service providers scrambled to meet the needs of an online-only society and began failing immediately. (Thurton, 2020) Faculty and students frantically searched for Internet providers able to install high-speed Internet where none existed. With libraries, community centers, restaurants, and cafes closed, there were few options to access Wi-Fi in the community. With a total population dependent on Internet access for every aspect of daily life, it was clear that existing Internet infrastructures were not capable of meeting the demand. No one anticipated a world in isolation due to a pandemic.

In 2020, Access Israel conducted a five-hour conference on inclusive remote education in response to a global lockdown due to the pandemic (Access Isreal, 2020). What emerged from that conference was a lack of paradigm shift from project-based inclusion to a cohesive action plan. For example, Huawei promoted portable Internet towers to provide service in Africa. However, this was presented as stand-alone proof of concept and not integrated with other accessible education solutions. Each "project" was presented as a stand-alone concept with no attempts to consolidate projects into a usable framework for accessible, inclusive learning. This solution would have been effective in the global north as well as the global south in alleviating the first gap in access to learning by people with disabilities. The focus would then have shifted to the Learning Management Systems and plethora of inaccessible content.

LEARNING MANAGEMENT SYSTEMS

If students managed to gain online access during the pandemic, they encountered Learning Management Systems (LMS) overwhelmed by a sudden need for every course to be offered online. An LMS is a digital classroom that, in many respects, attempts to mimic a bricks-and-mortar classroom experience for students and faculty.

While most brand-name LMSs have invested in accessibility for students with disabilities, most have not invested inaccessible interfaces and tools for faculty with disabilities. During the pandemic, teachers and students with disabilities faced barriers to teaching and learning.

Students were confronted with inaccessible elements of the LMS user interface followed by inaccessible course content. In some LMSs accessibility components are an additional cost or are considered a service which compounds barriers under normal circumstances. Academic institutions scrambled to confirm they had the accessibility components where the components were "add-ons". For those academic institutions where the academic institutions had switched LMSs in the fall of 2019, students had to learn the structure of a new LMS without access to support. At one college in Ontario, Canada, where the author lives, when asked about the accessibility of the new LMS, the IT department had to check to see if the accessibility components were purchased.

Even with legislation in most countries stating that an LMS must be accessible and that students with disabilities must be included in learning environments, this had not been happening at a pace that would support an academic system that had to shift within twenty-four hours to a learning environment solely based online. Additionally, most legislation does not include access to an LMS for faculty with disabilities. For example, the Integrated Accessibility Standards Regulations (IASR)2011 for Ontario Canada focuses on student access and doesn't mention access to LMSs or digital content for teachers or faculty (Government of Ontario, 2011).

ACCESS TO TEXTBOOKS

A lack of timely access to textbooks and course material creates another barrier to access to course content for students who are blind, have a visual learning or cognitive disability, have information processing issues, or have other types of print disabilities (Accessible Campus, 2018).

In monitoring the Assistive Technology in Higher Education Network (ATHEN) discussion group during the pandemic, the relationship between libraries, alternate text production centers, publishers, and students fell apart.

Those responsible for producing accessible versions of course material and textbooks found themselves working from home with none of the equipment they depended on to do their job. In alternate text production centers, there are high-speed scanners, the physical texts, machines to unbind textbooks for scanning, machines to rebind textbooks once they've been scanned, Optical Character Recognition (OCR or text recognition), adaptive technology for testing, and server access to store and distribute the learning material and textbooks. All of this infrastructure was removed overnight (ATHEN, 2020) when the decision was taken to work from home

Staff in alternate text production centres also order digital copies of textbooks that they then make accessible. There is a process and protocol in place for this and relationships with specific people at publishing companies. With the workforce on both sides of this equation scattered in their homes, the process faltered.

While articles estimate the shift toward digital textbooks increased during the pandemic (Ofgang, 2021 May), and the textbook industry embraced the change, there is no mention in any of the articles researched for this chapter that there is any attention being paid to ensuring the digital textbooks are accessible.

Publishers have one copy of a textbook but can produce three versions (print, PDF, and EPUB), two of them which are potentially accessible. The accessibility of textbooks and journals are dependent on the developer creating accessible InDesign documents to begin with. Adobe InDesign is the industry leader in desktop publishing software. InDesign provides document authors with the tools they need to create rich content with complex layouts and interactive elements for textbooks, magazines, brochures and almost all publishing needs (Adobe Systems, 2018). Adobe InDesign also has significant accessibility tools to convert accessible InDesign documents to accessible PDF or EPUB formats (Adobe Systems, 2018). For example, when someone is creating an InDesign document, they can add Alt text to images. This means that when someone using a screen reader or text-to-Speech tool comes across an image in either an accessible EPUB or tagged PDF document, they will be able to read the description (Alt Text) of the image.

In one of several articles on the rise of digital accessible textbooks, one student stated "they are open-minded tools". Accessible digital textbooks provide the same type of flexibility of learning that LMSs combined with face-to-face learning to learning does.

The goal for inclusive education is for all digital textbooks and journals to be mandated to be accessible and no digital textbook or journal is allowed to be used unless it is accessible (whether PDF or EPUB or any other format). This goal can be expanded to ensure that all portals used to access or purchase digital textbooks and journals are accessible so that students using adaptive technology can purchase or view accessible content.

COURSE CONTENT AND INCLUSION

A further goal toward inclusive education would be that while publishers trained staff to produce accessible content, tertiary level academic institutions would begin incorporating the design and creation of accessible digital content in all curricula within the learning environments as learning or course outcomes. If this important inclusion was made possible, it would be only a matter of time before anyone using any type of digital authoring tool would create digital content that is accessible by its very nature. In other words, digital content produced by graduates of tertiary academic institutions would be creating digital content, architecture and a built environment that would be "born accessible" and inclusive.

During the previous twenty years, some instructors have been hesitant to create accessible, inclusive content for courses (Lazar et al., 2011). Others had little or no experience teaching in a digital environment.

Instructors were plunged into online learning with little or no support as faculty instructional design staff scrambled to set up home computers to provide support. Even instructors with previous experience in online learning delivery had to find ways to provide captioning and other accessibility support for online conferencing software. One positive by-product of the pandemic was that the Zoom conferencing platform rapidly added captioning as did Microsoft Teams and both became competitors for academic decision-makers.

The inaccessibility of course content became the first barrier to be exposed as academic institutions discovered a plethora of content that was not accessible (Lazar J., 2022).

Faculty often choose tools not vetted for accessibility (Edmiston, 2013). Faculty looking for increased use of technology in the classroom often choose tools that are not accessible due to a lack of awareness of digital barriers. In an article on the rise of online learning during the pandemic, several LMSs were mentioned as providing free or low cost access to their services (Li, 2020). A search of the websites for the LMSs mentioned in the article resulted in no information about the accessibility of the LMS.

It was painfully obvious that the concept of unintentional barriers failed the test of time. There was no time to cajole faculty into creating accessible content for the greater good. Academic institutions had failed faculty and students with disabilities by not mandating inclusive education over the past twenty years.

During a discussion in a moderated accessibility list, one instructor stated that having students caption videos would be an unnecessary "burden" and that it was already a "burden" for academic institutions. During the pandemic, those in the conferencing software industry, aware of legislation and a human rights approach to education, moved to caption as a priority in their development roadmap and rose to the top of the list for academic institutions facing lawsuits for inaccessible online learning content. In 2021, UsableNet produced its annual report on digital accessibility. In their study, they sorted only lawsuits related to the inaccessibility of digital content. Their analysis shows an increase of 20% a year in the past four years of lawsuits in the United States specifically aimed at the inaccessibility of digital content (UsableNet, 2021).

An examination of the Ontario Ministry of Education website at the time of the pandemic, when the Ministry was directing K-12 teachers to use the TVO (Television Ontario) portal for learning, showed that little of the content was accessible to teachers and students with disabilities (AODA Alliance, 2020).

Advocates took to social media and conferencing tools. At that time, there was a four-to-five-month window of opportunity before the next wave of the pandemic struck (AODA Alliance, 2020). Globally, advocates were demanding the interval between pandemic waves not be wasted, and that strategy, plans, and actions commence (Australian Disability Clearinhouse on Education and Training, 2020). The author of this chapter reviewed plans for getting students in all learning systems back on campus in Canada and the United States and none addressed the lack of accessible content and identified clear strategies, policies, plans, and deadlines for inclusive education.

In June 2022, Mohawk College in Ontario Canada cancelled a "one-of-a-kind" Accessible Media Production graduate certificate program (Hristova, 2022) despite legislation to make Ontario accessible by 2025. The Integrated Accessibility Standards Regulations (IASR) identified the deadline of January 2021 for all public sector institutions, including the college, to be digitally accessible (Government of Ontario, 2011). This action illustrates the difficulty in "mandating" digital accessibility in academic institutions when staff and faculty learning opportunities are not present. A further complexity of the situation is the Equity, Diversity, and Inclusion Action Plan for the college (Mohawk College, 2022) which has several "commitments" to universal learning design, accessibility, and inclusion of people with disabilities in the community as well as the college.

As we emerge from the first pandemic of the digital age, the issue of mandating accessible digital content is evolving as a complex accessibility barrier. It is a sad commentary on the state of accessible digital design when, in 2022, a college has a "one-of-a-kind" accessible media program graduate certificate; that it is a "one-of-a-kind" and that it has been cancelled.

While there are some who believe that overnight we moved from thinking of accessibility as an ad hoc tool for individual students to recognizing that learning must be accessible by design (Anderson, 2020), the cancellation of an Accessible Media Production program graduate certificate illustrates a disconnect between the need and the reality. … As a community of tertiary academic institutions, we must find a way to provide a leadership role for the community, employers and our own students, staff and faculty.

STUDENT PARTICIPATION

The Ontario (Canada) government curriculum guides for secondary courses feature universal design as a component along with 'differentiated learning to meet the needs of students in Computer Studies (Government of Ontario, 2022) and in all subjects (Government of Ontario, 2022). The first accessibility barrier for students with disabilities is measuring the amount of accessible content developed by teachers in primary and secondary schools and how effective the teacher-training is in ensuring that digital content is accessible.

The second digital barrier is directly related to the experience of students with disabilities in online learning environments during a pandemic. While the flexibility of online learning may meet the needs of students with disabilities in their capacity to access learning material at any time, that learning material must be accessible (Heindel, 2014).

With most brand-name LMS incorporating accessibility as part of their product, students with disabilities encounter the same barriers they face in face-to-face learning. Faculty often lack disability awareness training. Faculty often don't understand the responsibilities of signing a commitment letter to provide reasonable accommodation. Communication between the faculty member and Disability Services is not collaborative (Heindel, 2014). When everyone is isolated in place, there is little room for flexibility in learning. Everything is remote with no opportunity for face-to-face or blended learning.

During the pandemic, students with disabilities were exponentially disconnected from their campus and the support needed to be successful in their academic careers (Anderson, 2020). Students with advocacy skills found it difficult to self-advocate due to the chaotic and fragmented structure of learning in a decentralized uncommunicative environment. While reports and articles on the retention rates of students with disabilities indicate that many left educations, it is only now that the pandemic is waning that we can truly examine the statistics and do a post-mortem on the level of failure of academic institutions toward faculty and students with disabilities.

Faculty and those working in alternate text production centers were trying to find free adaptive technology for students who no longer had access to technology that was licensed to bricks and mortar campuses (ATHEN, 2020). Once again, the limitations of enterprise license attached to a geographical point on a map from companies ill-equipped to shift to a new model of enterprise licensing failed students with disabilities. For example, students who had access to a screen reader on a campus computer but didn't have a screen reader on their home computer, were unable to access the campus license for the screen reader because the license was tied to the campus and not transferrable to off-campus access.

Without access to libraries, textbooks, accessible LMSs, and online content, many students were left behind. We know from World Bank and United Nations studies that for every year of education, an individual's income improves by about 10% (World Bank Group, 2022). It is not clear, now, whether students with disabilities left behind by an academic environment unwilling to enforce inclusion, will return to tertiary education soon or whether they will be a lost generation with unfulfilled life goals.

It is the accessibility of the LMS, combined with the accessibility of applications used in the course and the accessibility of the course content as well as all the partners in the learning process (faculty, librarians, Disability Services) that help break down the barriers to digital content for students with disabilities. Compartmentalization of the supports in a learning environment compounded by a pandemic contributes to digital barriers for students with disabilities.

CONCLUSION: ELIMINATING DIGITAL BARRIERS

Deanna Ferrante, a December graduate of the University of Massachusetts at Amherst, said in the article "Accessibility Suffers During Pandemic" that accessibility should not be framed as "guidelines" or "suggestions" for instructors but as a top-down mandate from university administrators' (Anderson, 2020). Accessibility and inclusion of faculty and students with disabilities at all levels of tertiary education should be a priority in 2022. In the same article by Anderson, Marion Quirici, a disability studies professor at Duke University said "Accessibility should be a 'state of mind,' and that has not historically been the case in higher education."

In most Tertiary level academic institutions, professional development and training opportunities for inclusive education are reverting to the status before the pandemic. This means that faculty are not mandated to produce accessible course content. The inclusion of students and other faculty in online learning environments is slipping back to only those who support inclusion. We are in danger of thinking of accessibility as an accommodation tool rather than an inclusive learning experience.

Some academic institutions have hired additional instructional designers with experience in inclusive design to work with faculty. As was the case before the pandemic, this service is often used by those who understand the need and ignored by those who don't.

Solutions to digital barriers have been present for several years: incorporating universal design, the WCAG POUR principles, and international standards of accessible digital environments and content in every aspect of the tertiary level policy, process, procurement, and delivery. From the top-down, there must be a process for identifying digital barriers and remediating them. This includes mechanisms for auditing and enforcement. There must be a clearly defined procurement process for any digital content, infrastructure, Learning Management System, anything digital must outline universal design principles, any legislative criteria around accessibility and any candidate for procurement must demonstrate that their product meets stringent criteria.

leadership and collaboration among tertiary-level academic institutions are key in moving toward the elimination of digital barriers. The procurement power of academic institutions must be leveraged to eliminate digital barriers. Leadership in inclusive education and inclusive digital environments must be proactive instead of reactive based on individual students and their needs. For example, ensuring that any video used in a course is captioned and video described eliminates the need for reasonable accommodation for students requiring those accessibility features. Ensuring a library portal/website is accessible making research material easier to locate by the student reduces the time staff spends helping students locate information.

Finally, support and funding for research projects into creating digital tools that adhere to universal design principles must be promoted within a collaborative tertiary-level academic institution system.

REFERENCES

Access Isreal. (2020, September 14). *Access Israel's 4th international webinar on "Inclusive Remote Education"*. Retrieved from Access Isreal https://www.aisrael.org/?CategoryID=2285&ArticleID=67270

Accessible Campus. (2018). *Understanding barriers to accessibility: An educator's perspective*. Retrieved from Council of Universities http://www.accessiblecampus.ca/tools-resources/educators-tool-kit/understanding-barriers-to-accessibility-an-educators-perspective/

Adobe Systems. (2018). *Adobe indesign accessibility training and resources*. Retrieved from Adobe Systems https://www.adobe.com/accessibility/products/indesign.html

Anderson, G. (2020, April 6). *Accessibility suffers during pandemic*. Retrieved from Inside Higher Ed: https://www.insidehighered.com/news/2020/04/06/remote-learning-shift-leaves-students-disabilities-behind

AODA Alliance. (2020, May 7). *The AODA alliance calls on TVO to take prompt action to fix its educational web contents accessibility problems*. Retrieved from AODA Alliance https://aoda.ca/the-aoda-alliance-calls-on-tvo-to-take-prompt-action-to-fix-its-educational-web-contents-accessibility-problems/

AODA Alliance. (2020, May 4). *Virtual townhall on students with disabilities during COVID*. Retrieved from https://www.youtube.com/watch?v=phdtibf5DbM: https://www.youtube.com/watch?v=phdtibf5DbM

ATHEN. (2020, 3). *March 2020 archives by subject*. Retrieved from Assistive Technology in Higher Education, University of Washington http://mailman12.u.washington.edu/pipermail/athen-list/2020-March/subject.html

Australian Disability Clearinghouse on Education and Training. (2020). *Podcast: ADCET crosses the ocean: Access & inclusion in Tertiary Education, Post-COVID-19 Part 3*. Retrieved from ADCET https://www.adcet.edu.au/resource/10347/podcast-adcet-crosses-the-ocean-access-inclusion-in-tertiary-education-post-covid-19-part-3

Edmiston, D. (2013, September 18). *20 Apps for academics in higher education*. Retrieved from The Marketing Prof.com: http://www.themarketingprof.com/higher-education-marketing/20-apps-academics-higher-education/

Government of Ontario. (2011, July 1). *Integrated accessibility standards regulations, Ontario regulation 191/11*. Retrieved from Government of Ontario, eLaws http://www.e-laws.gov.on.ca/html/regs/english/elaws_regs_110191_e.htm

Government of Ontario. (2022, June 8). *Cirriculum, secondary, by subject*. Retrieved from Ontario Government: http://www.edu.gov.on.ca/eng/curriculum/secondary/subjects.html

Government of Ontario. (2022, June 8). *Ontario curriculum: Computer studies, secondary*. Retrieved from https://www.dcp.edu.gov.on.ca/en/curriculum#secondary

Heindel, A. J. (2014, January 15). *A phenomenological study of the experiences of higher education students with disabilities*. Retrieved from University of South Florida, Scholar Commons, Graduate Theses and Dissertations extension://memepcobodlebmohdlfnjiaalggfcpic/https://digitalcommons.usf.edu/cgi/viewcontent.cgi?article=6233&context=etd

Hristova, B. (2022, June 9). *Mohawk College faces backlash for shuttering one-of-a-kind accessible media production program*. Retrieved from CBC (Canadian Broadcasting Corporation) https://www.cbc.ca/news/canada/hamilton/mohawk-college-accessible-media-production-program-1.6481612

Lazar, J., Goldstein, D., & Taylor, A. (2011). *Ensuring digital accessibility through process and policy*. Amsterdam, Holland: Elsevier Inc.

Lazar, J. (2022, June 8). *Managing digital accessibility at universities during the COVID-19 pandemic*. Retrieved from National Library of Medicine https://www.ncbi.nlm.nih.gov/pmc/articles/PMC7938369/

Li, C. (2020, April 27). *The COVID-19 pandemic has changed education forever. This is how*. Retrieved from Word Economic Forum: https://www.weforum.org/agenda/2020/04/coronavirus-education-global-covid19-online-digital-learning/

Mohawk College. (2022, June 10). *Equity, diversity and inclusion action plan*. Retrieved from Mohawk College https://www.mohawkcollege.ca/equity-diversity-and-inclusion

Ofgang, E. (2021, May 21). *Student Ebook reading surges during the pandemic*. Retrieved from Tech Learner https://www.techlearning.com/news/student-ebook-reading-surges-during-the-pandemic

Pulrang, A. (2021, March 21). *What disabled people are thinking and feeling about the pandemic, one year later*. Retrieved from Forbes https://www.forbes.com/sites/andrewpulrang/2021/03/21/what-disabled-people-are-thinking-and-feeling-about-the-pandemic-one-year-later/?sh=66e3f9093277

Thurton, D. (2020, May 25). *Pandemic drives demands for universal affordable internet and cell plans*. Retrieved from CBC News https://www.cbc.ca/news/politics/pandemic-covid-coronavirus-internet-cell-1.5581605

UsableNet. (2021, December 21). *2021 year end report – App & web accessibility lawsuits break records*. Retrieved from UsableNet https://blog.usablenet.com/2021-lawsuit-report-trends-and-findings#:~:text=The%20UsableNet%20research%20team%20monitors%20and%20documents%20all,The%20following%20report%20outlines%20trends%20found%20during%202021.

World Bank Group. (2022, May 1). *Education overview*. Retrieved from World Bank Group: https://www.worldbank.org/en/topic/education/overview#1

CHAPTER 20

Navigating the Mud of Tertiary Education: The Experience of Disabled Students at Universities in the Global South

TAFADZWA RUGOHO

INTRODUCTION

Zimbabwe witnessed a huge expansion in the 1990s and early 2000s in learning institutions that offer certificates, diplomas, degrees and other post-graduate qualifications to students, which also included students with disabilities. At Independence, Zimbabwe had one university, but now there are seven state universities, four universities established by Christian organizations and a women's university that are fully internationally accredited. In many of these institutions these students often face additional challenges and threats in their educational milieu (Rugoho & Jeffress, 2018). Students with disabilities face both physical and attitudinal barriers within their college or university environments. Attitudinal barriers are recognized widely as an impediment to success of people with disabilities (Rao, 2004).

In Zimbabwe, access to tertiary education for people with disabilities is seen as a privilege, not as a right. Students with disabilities are treated as charity cases and are not expected to excise any right in the selection of the degree programme they want. It is the prerogative of these universities to decide which programme suits the student. As a result of this practice, most students with disabilities are enrolled in arts and social science. Arts and social science are seen as easy subjects which students with disabilities are seen as having the capacity to cope with demands of these courses (Chiparaushe et al., 2011). Students with disabilities are rarely enrolled in science such as medicine, engineering, biology or mathematics.

Even faculties of Law Studies make it difficult for students with disabilities to enrol (Rugoho & Shumba, 2018).

I lost both legs below the knee when I was sixteen years old. I survived more than ten operations as doctors struggled to save my legs. The accident was so severe that I was hospitalised for close to two years. Soon after I had been discharged from the hospital, my parents began to arrange for me to go back to school. After years of struggling through the education system, I aimed for university education to enrol for a degree in law. At that time, law was only being offered at the University of Zimbabwe which is the largest university in the country. After failing to be enrolled for a law degree, I was literally offered to study sociology. However, the university did not specify the reasons I was not awarded an opportunity to study law. After finishing my sociology degree, I later went for two master's degrees in sociology in other two separate universities. During my years at university, I faced many challenges.

This chapter will discuss the challenges faced by students with disabilities in the universities. While focussing on Zimbabwe, it will recommend what should be done by the universities in the global south to improve the learning environment for people with disabilities. For those institutions, the chapter offers strategies that will enhance inclusion of people with disabilities. In this chapter, I argue that choice of study must be expanded and highlight the need for policies that enshrine the inclusion of students with disabilities in tertiary education. When I was writing this chapter, I was enrolled at two different universities. One in a developing country and the other at developed country. At both universities I was enrolled for doctoral studies. While my own experience guides this discussion, it is backed by current literature highlighting those areas needing improvement and those attitudes that need changing.

Students with disabilities face mammoth tasks when enrolling at universities in Zimbabwe (Chataika et al., 2012). This is because universities are poorly prepared to accommodate students with disabilities (Chireshe, 2013). Staff at universities often lacks awareness on disability (Lyner-Cleophas et al., 2014). When I arrived at the university I faced many challenges. On the day I went to get my application form I went with a wheelchair. The first thing I faced were the physical barriers. There were a lot of steps to use when getting to offices on higher floors and there were no provisions of elevators. The admission forms were on the second floor of the building. There were no elevators.

CHOICE OF DEGREE PROGRAMMES

Graduation records from Zimbabwe's University Disability Resource Centres show that the majority of people with disabilities with degrees have graduated from the Faculties of Arts (Rugoho & Shumba, 2018). When I enrolled as an undergraduate, a large population of students with disabilities were enrolled in the Arts departments. Some were enrolled in Faculties of Social Sciences pursuing degrees in political science, sociology and administration. Very few were enrolled in social work and law. On rare occasions, you would see a student with disabilities enrolled in natural sciences. Universities in Zimbabwe rarely allow students with disabilities to enrol in the physical science (Rugoho & Shumba, 2018). As a result, students with disabilities face challenges in getting employment after finishing their degrees because they enrolled in majors which have less marketability (Chiparaushe et al., 2011).

Students with disabilities are not given the option to choose the degree of their choice; most are usually offered what they can study by the university. During the course of my studies, I noticed that the majority of students, especially those in arts degrees, were forced to take up those programs. These degrees were never their choices. Universities use the points score criteria to allocate degrees. Those with higher points at Advanced Level (the General Certificate of Education, or GCE) are allocated degrees in physical sciences, business and law if they do not have a disability. In some instances, the criteria are also used to students with disabilities regardless of their situations. Going to school with a disability can be difficult. Students with disabilities face multiple challenges which also make it hard to score higher points. Some schools do not have resources, especially for visually impaired students. The inaccessible learning environment hinders those with disabilities from reaching higher academic achievement. Universities should be able to understand these challenges and allow students with disabilities to enrol in courses of our choices. Departments need to provide opportunities and resources to assist students with disabilities. One of my friends with cerebral palsy who had scored higher points and qualified to enrol for medicine was told by the chairperson:

> We can't enrol you for medicine because of your condition. How would you cope in the lab? You will not only be a danger to yourself but to others as well. I don't think there would be any patient that would want to be treated by you. Just go and enrol in the faculty of arts where other students with disabilities are enrolled. Here, we can't give you a place. (Rugoho, in press)

CHALLENGES IN PHYSICAL ACCESS

One of the greatest challenges faced by students with disabilities within higher education is physical access. Universities in Zimbabwe have not yet adjusted their infrastructure to be accessible for people with disabilities. Many physical challenges still exist. Lecture rooms have steps and many do not have elevators (Obiozor, 2011). Although accessibility has been improved considerably during the past decade through the use of automatic doors, ramps, and lifts for those with restricted mobility, many of those doors are still not wide enough for electric wheel chairs limiting access to auditoria and laboratories. One of the most common complaints of physically disabled people is the inaccessibility of the environment caused by architectural barriers (Rugoho & Shumba, 2018).

Attitudinal barriers are considered much worse than architectural barriers. There might be a ramp to a stage of the theatre, but their policy does not allow students with mobility impairments to audition for a play (Rugoho & Shumba, 2018). Attitudinal issues are the most significant barrier to progress (Rugoho & Jeffress, 2018). Negative attitudes towards students with disabilities may result in low acceptance by peers, limited friendships, loneliness and even being rejected or bullied (Shetgiri, 2013).

Institutions need to consider the unique challenges that are faced by their students (Obiozor, 2011). While a lecture may be conveyed in a venue in the second or third floor of buildings, administrators of the faculty must be aware that these physical environments do not have elevators. How would students on wheelchairs get to these venues? If the lecturer proceeds before the department administrator is looking for an optional venue, the student with a disability will be left behind. While I was in my second year of study, members of the class who were disabled were at one time forced to seek the intervention of the departmental chair after the lecturer refused to change location, citing that there is no alternative venue. Looking for a proper venue through confrontation, students with disabilities may appear to have enmity towards their lecturers, even though they simply asked for access to learning. Some lecturers may see this as challenging their authority and possibly form a negative attitude towards students with disabilities. When I was still a student, I had to be diplomatic with the lecturers so that they understand our challenges when it comes to accessibility. Once, I went to church where one of the lecturers attends and presented our issues to the lecturer in front of her pastor soon after the church service ended. I was surprised that she (paster) understood me better. Deep down I knew she wanted to please her pastor, but for me it was a mission accomplished.

Deaf students also face communication barriers in lecture room and other areas at the university. During my undergraduate studies Deaf students took similar courses with me. Lectures were delivered in spoken English. The university did not employ a sign language interpreter and Deaf students were forced to read the lips of their lecturers. Tutorials are compulsory, and Deaf students were forced to attend to and gaze at other people—as no accommodations were offered. A fellow Deaf student put it candidly:

This is torture of the highest level. We are not benefiting from these lecturers and tutorials. How would they have felt if they were in my position? Imagine being forced to sit and watch something that you do not even understand. I have wasted my time enrolling at this university. It was better for me to do distance education. The university does not understand that we are not benefiting. I can't even express how I feel to the chairperson. He does not understand me. When he sees me in his office his facial expressions clearly tells me that I am not welcome. However, as outcasts we have to play by their rules. (Rugoho, in press)

TECHNOLOGICAL CHALLENGES

Access to information does not only affect Deaf students, but students with visual impairments as well. In Zimbabwe, the majority of visually impaired students rely on another person to read for them—a model of dependency that frequently creates barriers. In some cases, reading material is recorded using tape recorders, which allows the visually impaired person to listen to whenever she/he wants. This is the most wide spread practice in most colleges, schools, and some universities (Chiparaushe et al., 2011). Students rely on donated tape recorders and cassette players. The recordings are done by volunteers who are not professionals, therefore recordings may have defects, making it hard for visually impaired people to clearly grasp everything that is recorded. Diagrams and illustrations in the text cannot be captured by recordings.

However, with electronic reader software, technology navigation is very easy, and offers independence for users. It has the capacity to refer the reader to the chapter or subtopic that they would want to read. This is different with books recorded by tape recorders, which is difficult to locate subtopics that they are interested in listening to. There are a number of software programs, such as Job Access with Speech (JAWS). JAWS is a computer screen reader program for Microsoft Windows that allows blind and visually impaired users to read the screen either with a text-to-speech output or by a refreshable Braille display. A visually impaired student said:

All that is needed is commitment on the part of the institutions. It is a good resource—I use it myself. But it has a considerable financial cost. You might acknowledge this here. (Rugoho, in press)

Smart technology is being adopted by institutions in higher education worldwide. Smart technology has the potential to improve access and the quality of education for disabled people (Firmin et al., 2013). Smart education allows students to utilize technological devices to access digital resources through wireless networks and to immerse in both personalized and seamless learning. It has also facilitated students to learn more effectively, efficiently, flexibly and comfortably

(Zhu et al., 2016). Smart education has the potential to address the challenges of the 21st century and provide flexibility in the mode of learning (Zhu et al., 2016). Unfortunately, universities in Zimbabwe have not yet fully embraced it (Rugoho & Shumba, 2018).

SPORTING AND SOCIAL CHALLENGES

Sporting activities have the potential to foster greater inclusion and well-being for persons with disabilities (Dada & Ukpata, 2017). At the university where I enrolled for my undergraduate studies, we tried a number of initiatives to be included at sporting activities, but the sports director seemed to have little understanding about how people with disabilities could participate. Instead of taking a responsibility, he shifted that to the Disability Resource Centre staff who were supposed to help with our academic and campus challenges.

Only after lobbying and advocating, we were able to participate in national competitions. The assistance that we managed to get from the university was meagre. We had to approach donors for funding. While the university had budgets for sporting activities, the university did not have a disability policy on how students with disabilities were to be supported and included. Our participation in other sporting activities were dependant on the benevolence of the Vice Chancellor, or other stakeholders. In the other universities I latter enrolled in, I noticed that students with disabilities were not included in sporting activities. Universities need to not only develop policies on the inclusion of students with disabilities in sport activities, but also facilitate and fund sports clubs to include students with disabilities. Universities can also consider giving sporting scholarships to students with disabilities.

OVERCOMING CHALLENGES FACING DISABLED PEOPLE IN HIGHER EDUCATION IN THE GLOBAL SOUTH

While the number of students with disabilities in higher education is increasing, the experience of students with disabilities at university campuses is not improving. Universities need to improve their infrastructure to make sure that it is accessible. Students face challenges in accessing pivotal places such as lecture rooms and libraries. They cannot learn if they cannot access the place of learning.

Universities need to be innovative learning centres where all students can maximize their potential. By adopting modern technology, students with disabilities can become more independent in their studies. Universities must strive to improve on all the rights of people with disabilities.

Universities across the southern world must draw from their existing official disability policies that clearly spell out rights and provisions for those with disabilities. Activists must continue to advocate for the inclusion of people with disabilities by reducing institutional, environmental and personal attitudinal barriers. Universities must join with them and become a leading force for change.

Students with disabilities at universities also need to collaborate to push for improvement that affects their rights. As seen in most universities and colleges in developing countries, students with disabilities do not have organisations that represent themselves. Most institutions take advantage of this disorganisation and remain irresponsible for improving students' welfare and disability rights. Further, students need to understand university policies, national laws, and international treaties on disability to which their countries should adhere. This will help in bringing litigation against universities.

Social media is another way students with disabilities should utilise to spread awareness and advocate for the implementation of their rights in colleges and universities. Most minority groups in the world are using social media to lobby and advocate. Students with disabilities should show the state of these universities to the world to encourage university administrations and the ministers to take more responsibility.

REFERENCES

Chataika, T., Mckenzie, J. A., Swart, E., & Lyner-Cleophas, M. (2012). Access to education in Africa: Responding to the United Nations convention on the rights of persons with disabilities. *Disability & Society*, *27*(3), 385–398.

Chiparaushe, B., Mapako, O., & Makarau, A. (2011). *A survey of challenges, opportunities and threats faced by students with disabilities in the post independent era in Zimbabwe*. Harare, Zimbabwe: Students Solidarity Trust.

Chireshe, R. (2013). The state of inclusive education in Zimbabwe: Bachelor of education (special needs education) students' perception. *Journal of Social Science*, *34*(3), 223–228.

Dada, O. A., & Ukpata, C. O. (2017). Sport participation and facilities as predictors of marketable skills in sport for persons with disability in Nigerian Universities. *European Journal of Special Education Research*, *2*(5), 135–146.

Firmin, M. W., Firmin, R. L., & Merical, K. L. (2013). Extended communication efforts involved with college long-distance relationships. *Contemporary Issues in Education Research*, *6*(1), 97–110.

Lyner-Cleophas, M., Swart, E., Chataika, T., & Bell, D. (2014). Increasing access into higher education: Insights from the 2011 African Network on Evidence-to-Action on Disability Symposium—Education Commission. *African Journal of Disability*, *3*(2), 1–11.

Obiozor, W. E. (2011). Literacy and social challenges facing exceptional students: A discourse on higher institutions experience in America and lessons for African societies. In R. L. Dalla, O. Okeke, & A. T. Ahon, *Education in contemporary perspectives* (pp. 67–89). Abuja, Nigeria: Fab Educational Publishers.

Rao, S. (2004). Faculty attitudes and students with disabilities in higher education: A literature review. *College Student Journal, 38*(2), 191–198.

Rugoho, T. (2019). My disability, my ammunition, my asset. In Berghs, Maria and Chataika, Tsitsi (Eds.), *Routledge handbook on disability activism*. London, UK: Routledge.

Rugoho, T., & Jeffress, M. S. (2018). My class, my disability, my struggle. In M. S. Jeffress (Ed.), *International perspectives on teaching with disability: Overcoming obstacles and enriching lives* (pp. 50–61). London, UK: Routledge.

Rugoho, T., & Shumba, J. (2018). Disabled refugee students in Zimbabwe. In S. Enakshi & P. Blessinger (Eds.), *Refugee education: Strategies, policies and directions* (pp. 117–128). London, UK: Emerald Group Publishing.

Shetgiri, R. (2013). Bullying and victimization among Children. *Advances in Pediatrics, 60*(1), 33–51.

Zhu, Z., Yu, M. H., & Riezebos, P. (2016). A research framework of smart education. *Smart Learning Environments, 2*(9), 1–17.

CHAPTER 21

Even the Delusional Can Learn: The Recognition of Diverse States of Mind, Knowing and Being

MAREE ROCHE

> When I am at my present "normal" self I am far removed from when I have been my liveliest, most productive, most intense, most outgoing and effervescent. In short, for myself, I am a hard act to follow. (Kay Redfield Jamison, 1997, p. 92)

INTRODUCTION

I was astounded when I applied for (and successfully attained) postgraduate entry, complete with a university funded scholarship, five years after I was diagnosed with Bipolar Disorder. I had spent the years between diagnosis to admission wondering if I had the capacity to learn, to create and to excel in an area that seemed to be only for the well and ably minded. My mind, as far as I was concerned, was different; and by different I meant not "normal." Would I be able to fit into the institution? More importantly, would I be acknowledged, understood and supported?

Generally, Bipolar Disorder is the term used to describe a set of "mood swinging" behaviours. It usually incorporates swings related to emotions, cognition, reactions and energy from one extreme to the other, from incredible euphoria and the bleakest lows. One of the characteristics of Bipolar Type I Disorder, as opposed to Type II, is mania and the manic "highs." Mania is associated with elevated moods, feeling invincible, and creativity mixed with impulsive behaviour.

For university students, it could involve not sleeping for a few days yet still feeling energised and being able to complete work at the last minute. It could also mean an abundance of grandiose ideas filled with much enthusiasm on group assignments, feeling over confident, super excited and engaging in inappropriate behaviour. Conversely, Depression in Bipolar Type 1 for university students may lead to feelings of worthlessness in the quality of work being produced, inactivity and lethargy (unable or have the want to finish assessments) difficulty concentrating and understanding the work, and wanting to drop out of university because it feels too hard and too cumbersome.

When elevated—not able to sit still, frequent talking in rapid speech, heightened verbosity, ideas flowing—can impact fellow students as they may find it difficult to keep up or fully understand. Lecturers may also be uncertain as to what the student is trying to communicate through their written work or unit presentations. This can affect relationships, both in group settings and personal circumstances, as well as learning and responding to rigid assessment criteria.

It is essential that within the institution itself, administration creates a positive learning environment that is reflective of diversity and equity. While each student can develop and employ strategies for studying with complex mental health challenges, the onus need not fall on to the student to fit into a specific model. If the model had inbuilt flexibility, variety of supports, acknowledgements and adaptability, the university experience could cater to the student's individual needs.

This chapter argues that institutions need to acknowledge and validate psychosocial disabilities and the capacity in which students can learn. It challenges the bio-psycho-social account of specificity relating the "mental capacity" required to undertake university study, and the institutional capital of higher education providers whose remit is to include any number of "equity groups" to access degree-level qualifications while at the same time tacitly placating their admission. Increasing numbers of university students are experiencing mental health challenges with many escalating in severity. Anxiety and depression can be seen to be serious issues at US universities; over 40% of students surveyed by the American College Health Association reported that they were so depressed at times that it was difficult for them to function (Reilly, 2018). In the UK, the rate of students experiencing mental ill health having to discontinue their courses increased 210% over a five-year period (Baron, 2017).

What differentiates complex mental health challenges from physical disabilities is temporality. Mental health challenges are not always fixed and instead can be episodic. There are fluctuating periods on which quality learning can take place within and without those challenges. Much of my postgraduate learning occurred online, away from the physicality, noise and business of a bricks and mortar campus—the machinations and routines that can be liked to an elevated mood that feels like mania. The online environment provided the opportunity to undertake university studies without the anxiety driven compulsion of mandatory participation of class times, lectures and what I like to term, "people-ling." The online environment also provided an equitable way of completing studies without the additional challenges of what a physical classroom and wider campus environment may present. What is present in this chapter as "multi modal" learning is an approach that can make further study a possibility for more students with complex mental health challenges. Universities must change the delivery and structure of their courses and their approaches to teaching to include student voice through the co-production of strategies, techniques and resources that can benefit all students.

HIGH VOLTAGE THINKING, SLUDGE AND SLURRY

> Who would not want an illness that has among its symptoms elevated and expansive mood, inflated self-esteem, abundance of energy, less need for sleep, intensified sexuality …. —Kay Redfield Jamison (1994, p. 103)

Learning & Studying During a Hypo/Manic Episode

There is a euphoric kind of exhilaration and creativity that oftentimes arrives with a manic episode. Ideas are rapidly flowing, thoughts are fizzing over with excitement and inspiration is as expansive as it is accelerating. Some of my best academic work was completed during those manic episodes. I seemed to have an ability to push past what I perceived to be deficient thinking and reach a new area of in-depth analysis and new, unseen discoveries. My mind was focused and clear and everything finally made sense. All seemed to fit within the universe. Life was just superb, albeit fast! However, with high voltage thinking also comes high voltage collateral damage. With mania also comes recklessness, poor judgement, frenetic and incomprehensible behaviour. Many times, it may be difficult to remember the full scope of what happened during that episode. Information that was easy to read might later be considered unintelligible and difficult, no matter how many times it is read.

Within the first trimester of my postgraduate studies I had tipped into a manic episode, partly owing to excitement and partly owing to the terrifying fear of failure. I initially struggled with disclosure and felt that even though I was a student with a scholarship, I was an imposter, and this manic episode that threatened to undo all my "good work" was either going to ruin me or shoot my successes into stardom. I could either drop out of university or I could work out a way in which I was able to successfully study and thrive with all the fragmented parts that kept me together.

The decision to disclose to lecturers and or supervisors while in a manic episode is a problematic one. One of the biggest issues for me was my own self-imposed stigma associated with bipolar disorder and complex mental health challenges overall. I was also preoccupied about what others may think I was able and unable to do.

Disclosing allowed my supervisor to put the copious number of e-mails that I have sent into context. I also let my supervisor know because it is important to have people we can trust academically to advocate and support when we ask for it or need it. It is empowering, as what may be considered delightful, can indeed be erratic and confusing. Unfortunately, it is very rare to find a university support system that deals with the practicalities and studying through episodes, other than counselling services that provide support on an emotional and psychological level. A learning support plan from the disability support services on campus may also assist in implementing certain strategies during periods of unwellness.

Self-awareness and insight are the foundation of any study plan. While in a manic episode I learned to write questions down in a word processing document to revise or revisit later. If I was compelled to talk to my supervisor or lecturer/professor and share my wonderful ideas, I learned to do so via e-mail and hit the "save to draft" function rather than send it off. That way, I could reconsider those ideas after the manic episode and work out what was good (there may actually be a lot of ideas that are!) and what may be not so practical or coherent. I learned to break assignments into paragraphs and have a couple of browser windows open. I also saved my work to an online cloud space to ensure consistency if I was working on multiple devices. This allowed me to share my work for ongoing corrections and comments. As ideas swing from one assignment to another, I would jot them down. This enables my attention (even though it may be swinging) to go back to the task by working towards the assignment.

Decreased need for sleep in mania can be considered both a symptom and a cause, in that not wanting to sleep is an indicator of a potential manic episode, while not sleeping can cause a manic episode. Sleep is important. When ideas pop into the head at three in the morning with an overwhelming compulsion to write an assignment right there and then, a paper journal or notebook by the bedside helped. Sometimes I used my smartphone as a voice recorder to quickly and securely get the thought out of my mind and return to sleep. During these times I often advised my lecturer should I be late to an online forum meeting because I slept in or was not feeling up to heavy learning. That way, I gained control of my learning and those around me were able to help put supports in place to ensure that I could perform at my best.

As a result of sleep disruption or even an adjustment to medication, it can be hard to focus, especially if accompanied by agitation and irritability. Only through flexibility in the model of course delivery was I able to complete my course of study. When it was too difficult to concentrate during class time, I was able to arrange to complete some of the class within the allotted time frame and some later.

Can the student sit in an additional tutorial or obtain the lecture online or via a podcast? Can the student break their day into manageable chunks? Multiple enrolment formats allow students to attend classes both in person and online and supports multi-modal enrolment. Multi-modal, in essence, refers to communication or learning undertaken in combinations of two or more modes. Students are able to learn effectively during episodes and make meaning of what they are learning. However, this requires universities to provide education across diverse and equitable forms.

Learning and Studying during a Depressive Episode

During a depressive episode, crawling out from under the blankets, let alone leaving the house, is a Herculean feat. Pretending I was well when I felt miserable and incapable is how I began my second trimester at university. Depression applied to learning, for many, consists of lethargy, apathy, sleep disturbance, self-blame, worthlessness, impaired memory and concentration, anxiety and loss of pleasure and enjoyment. Material learning in class, which during a manic episode was exciting and easy to understand, during a depressive episode can be incoherent. Instead of reading textbooks I would stare outside the window wondering why what I used to be able to study faultlessly is now such a struggle. The course I once started with high hopes and intentions became dull, lifeless and meaningless with a heavy dose of tiredness and restlessness. I also became mistrustful and weary as to who I could express my concerns to. Talking about complex mental health challenges at university is a selective business.

During a depressive episode dealing with people can sometimes be difficult when there are assignments to complete. Clearing the calendar and prioritising can mean that the student could look after themselves, and complete assessments at a pace they are comfortable with. Hanging up the "do not disturb" sign on the door can take the pressure of trying to keep up with the daily demands and the guilt that can arise compounds feelings that are already bringing them down. If allowed to work at their own pace, in their own time, much of this pressure can be alleviated. This is about how the course can fit in with the needs of the student, or at least meeting the student half way. By adapting the approach, learning can still occur in diverse states of mind and being.

WHAT DO STUDENTS NEED?

Although students may have similar mental health challenges, they are unique to the individual. This is critical as institutions are required to ensure that students with mental health challenges are able to access and participate in education on the same basis as other students, in accordance with the disability legislation.

The first step to equitable learning and inclusion is a deep understanding and a confident, well-informed response to the mental health challenges of students. Institutions can assist their academic and administrative staff by supporting attendance to relevant workshops on mental health and equip them with sound knowledge and skills when students self-disclose or may present to class during an episode. Sound information and strategies surrounding disclosure and challenges should also be made widely available to all university students as not all students may have received an official diagnosis. This will allow students to feel secure and safe to approach faculty or administration without feeling as though there may not be a resolution or are "left hanging" with no compassion, understanding or pathways. Disclosure for the student can be a tricky business as the outcomes are not always predictable. Providing positive, warm and safe predictability will guide the student towards success.

It is essential to determine adjustments with the student co-productively as a preventative measure, and also during an episode. This allows institutions, and in particular, academics to adjust their assessments equitably. This also permits institutions to become present in their student's educational experiences and better understand the warning signs and strategies needed to ensure equitable university success. The success presented in inclusive communication draws upon the knowledge of staff and validates student strengths while acknowledging the mental health challenges that are involved with university study.

Physical accessibility to higher education for a student with a mental health challenge can be considered vastly different from students with a physical or noticed disability. There are many factors that may contribute to elevated mood and heightened anxiety that present barriers to accessibility: large crowds, bright lighting, multiple conversations and the large information transference within a short amount of time. For students with mental health issues, there may be times when dealing with people can be difficult in a class/group work situation owing to anxieties or sensory distortion. Sounds may seem louder or sharper, colours brighter, touch unexpected, smells more pungent. Sometimes objects become distorted or frightening (Deveson, 1998).

Institutions need to consider a delivery model that allows students to participate in online and on-campus classrooms. Multimodal learning environments allow instructional elements to be presented in more than one sensory mode (visual, aural, written) (Sankey et al., 2010). Taking this one step further, this approach can be applied to subject flexibility for continued and successful learning throughout episodes allowing universities to innovate beyond the notion that they "still privilege certain ways of knowing and focus on a narrow view of the intellect that does not always allow for socio-cultural differences" (Barrington, 2004, p. 422).

The online environment can be particularly useful when external stimuli interferes with concentration. By developing and providing multi-modal options, continued learning will be made possible. This flexibility provides a continuum allowing the student to engage on an equitable level with other students in their diverse state of mind. It also considers how learning choices fulfil the purpose of studying, the students' abilities within the context of mental challenges, and how those modes work together in the development of knowing, learning and equitable education. Doing so validates the mental health challenges as diversity and provides opportunities for all students to learn.

REFERENCES

Baron, E. (2017). Eleven sketches inspired by the university mental health crisis—in pictures. *The Guardian*. Retrieved from https://www.theguardian.com/education/gallery/2017/jun/27/eleven-sketches-university-mental-health-crisis>

Barrington, E. (2004). Teaching to student diversity in higher education: How multiple intelligence theory can help. *Teaching in Higher Education, 9*(4), 421–434.

Deveson, A. (1998). *Tell me I'm here* (2nd ed.). Sidney, Australia: Penguin Books.

Jamison, K. R. (1994). *Touched with fire: Manic-depressive illness and the artistic temperament*. New York, NY: Simon & Schuster.

Jamison, K. R. (1997). *The Unquiet Mind: A memoir of moods and madness*. London, UK: Picador.

Reilly, K. (2018). Record numbers of college students are seeking treatment for depression and anxiety—But schools can't keep up. *Time Magazine*. Retrieved from http://time.com/5190291/anxiety-depression-college-university-students/

Sankey, M., Birch, D., & Gardiner, M. (2010). Engaging students through multimodal learning environments: The journey continues. In C. H. Steel, M. J. Keppell, P. Gerbic, & S. Housego (Eds.), *Curriculum, technology & transformation for an unknown future* (pp. 852–863).

CHAPTER 22

From Classification to Culture: Learning Disabilities in Higher Education

MATTHEW BEREZA

INTRODUCTION

Most of my life I have struggled against a pressure to remain quiet about the learning disability that affects my reading and writing. I was unable to keep up with my peers in school and was publicly singled out for not being able to perform at grade level. At a young age I did not know what was happening to me, or why I was so confused when reading or writing. I could not express this frustration to teachers, I only knew that my classmates were completing assignments I could not. Early in my life I knew I did not want to fail, I only wanted to be like other kids who remained in their "mainstream" classrooms all day. Mostly, I did not want to be different from my friends and have to do "special" assignments. Instead, I gave into torpor. Torpor is the tendency to view a situation as unchangeable (Martin-Baró, 1994). Torpor has a heavy gravitational pull, where failure is not a possibility, but an expectation. Regardless, I did go on to complete school and eventually earned a doctoral degree in the sciences. It was a struggle, at times unnecessarily, and my disability was always present. During those years I learned that no one is going to hand a learning-disabled student a degree, they have to struggle in ways that others do not.

This chapter speaks to learning disabled students who want a college education. This chapter also speaks to higher education providers, advocating for competent disability assistance and education on campuses so we may succeed.

To prospective students, I advocate for linking up with any available resources upon arrival at the university, and I detail how my experiences in the assistive learning laboratory became not only "assistive," but social. I also challenge disabled students to come together to create a recognizable culture on campus, allying with groups who have had success changing higher education. This culture, and buy-in from universities, is what will change higher education into a place for everyone.

This chapter also calls for higher education providers to provide competent disability assistance and education on campus so students with learning disabilities may succeed. While there are universities offering adequate services and embracing students with disabilities, too many do not. Even more troubling is the lingering stigma surrounding learning disability, and a view that students with learning disabilities pose a risk for scholarship in higher education. Throughout my time as a student with learning difficulties, as a graduate assistant, and as a licensed educational psychologist, I have seen what works and what is missing. In this chapter I argue for more services based on the needs of individual students. Without this investment, higher education will continue to lose countless students to a vague and unfounded belief that they do not belong in post-school education.

Ultimately, this chapter envisions a campus where learning disabled students stand equal among the various cultures and groups. To understand this vision, we must look to theory and how student struggles have defined experience.

LET THEORY AND PRACTICE DEFINE DISABILITY

Perhaps the most elegant definition of a learning disability is "to struggle" (Pelkey, 2001). In this chapter learning disability is seen as part of an enduring *culture,* instead of a temporary handicap on the way to the perceived freedoms of able-bodiedness. Some define disability culture using Crip Theory (McRuer, 2006). Crip Theory takes into account essential aspects of Queer Theory, Feminism, and Critical Theory while questioning whether individuals with disabilities should even seek to be included in oppressive systems as they currently exist. Instead, these paradigms call for a transformation of structured services, such as mainstream education. Disability, through these orientations, becomes a culture in its own right, not a failing. Crip Theory and Liberation Psychology (Martin-Baró, 1994) point to ways that learning-disabled students can question entrenched structures and struggle for justice in education. As a result of reimagining their lives, and with universities dedicating resources to learning disabilities, students can co-create that which has not come before: A new culture on campus.

There are barriers to this process. Universities in the U.S. and elsewhere enjoy near-exemption from laws requiring them to identify students with learning disabilities. If a university student has previously been classified with a disability, they may submit documentation while studying at the university and have limited protections under the Americans with Disabilities Act (ADA) (Sparks & Lovett, 2014). The ADA, however, has a clause requiring students to demonstrate how a disability substantially limits one or more major life activities. In addition, if an accommodation is financially or structurally unreasonable for a university to implement, it can be denied and the disabled student must fend for themselves. This may explain why so many smaller institutions offer limited and inexpensive accommodations, such as extended time on assignments and tutoring (Tzivinikou, 2014). To compound the issue, over half of universities polled utilize the discrepancy model between intelligence and ability (Madaus et al., 2010). The discrepancy model assumes that all students should achieve at nearly the same level, and if they cannot, they are labeled learning disabled. Many of the instruments used in the discrepancy model are based on dominant-cultural norms and do not measure how a student responds to personalized interventions. These tests must be administered by a licensed professional and can be a time and financial burden upon the learning-disabled student.

As a result, the lack of progressive and innovative interventions has been a disservice to unique learners, leaving the responsibility of navigating unfriendly and imposing environments (i.e., the university) upon the individual. Throughout my experience as a learning disability services graduate assistant, I played a part in this machine: I tested and measured students—detailing their strengths, weaknesses, and educational/career aspirations. These students would often present to my office with thick folders of documentation and carefully planned interventions, and we would vigorously analyze them. Unfortunately, the majority of accommodations granted by the university were limited to completing tests in a quiet environment and extra tutoring. In many ways, higher education was taking the path of least resistance by not adequately investing in support services and laboratories for learning disabled students. Ultimately, it became clear that higher education providers gravitate to the argument that they do not have time to individualize education (Walker, 2016). The message is unmistakable: disabled students must accept mainstream education through inclusion.

Inclusion, if correctly implemented, describes how "mainstream" institutions work toward the continuity of disabled students in a desired environment (Morgado et al., 2016). The understanding of inclusion in higher education is confused, and elicits uncomfortable questions as to why disabled students must change parts of their culture. While faculty and mainstream education students are favorable about having students with a disability in class, and report having significant exposure to them, they are not recruited as other *cultures* (Gibbons et al., 2015).

Radical Inclusion (Greenstein, 2015) is a model that higher education must adopt to transform. Radical Inclusion demands disability is accepted as political rather than medical, and sees us in the process of becoming in the world with others (Oliver, 2009). An analogy of this process occurs in gender studies in the "coming out" process. Mainstream disability culture is largely defined by compulsory able-bodiedness and normative lifestyles (McRuer, 2006) and carries strict norms that are placed upon disability. The process of discovering and accepting gender (or learning style) is a deeply personal one and belongs solely to the individual. No one or institution has the power to dictate what people are and when and how they will disclose our identity.

The same is true for the learning-disabled student. The process of exploration, acceptance, and coming out with a learning disability must be fostered and honored. When and how they complete this journey must also be safely settled in the individual, not the institution. Just as higher education has come to accept (in many cases) gender exploration and rights, it needs to do so in terms of learning disabilities. Higher education can embrace this radical approach of disability as a culture by deeply getting to know their students. This will take work as learning-disabled culture celebrates itself in nontraditional ways that often are at odds with higher education.

STRATEGIES FOR UNIVERSITY STUDENTS WITH LEARNING DISABILITIES

A guiding principle for students with learning disabilities attempting university education is to challenge any beliefs that control or hide your disability. When I entered university, I believed my disability would evaporate and I would bloom in the supportive and challenging atmosphere of higher education. Nothing could have been further from the truth, and I nearly failed my first semester. I later realized that the sooner disabled students link up with support services such as a mentor, the longer they stay in the university (Chambliss & Takacs, 2014). This could be as easy as disclosing your disability to your advisor the first week of school or trusting a professional in the university. Be creative in this search for allies, and gauge any prejudices carefully, as many universities simply do not have dedicated and "brightly lit" environments for learning disabled students. It is your responsibility to expand your search on campus and in the surrounding community. If the university offers services, start there, but if not, seek out campus members who demonstrate progressive ideas. As an undergraduate student, I found an assistant librarian and the school's minister to be incredibly important supports, even though I didn't initially consider them as potential allies. I was attracted to them because I heard about their work in social justice issues on campus.

Link up with the university's office for disability services the first week of class and ask if they have an assistive technology laboratory. This laboratory is much more than a place to complete assignments, it is where other students with disabilities will be found. Explore these labs, if the university offers one, and become acquainted with the people who work there as they may be disabled and know how to navigate higher educational structures. These relationships helped me break down the limitations I had placed upon myself struggling in isolation. By meeting other disabled students, I grew socially and academically without the monitoring of mainstream educators and administrators. Another benefit of becoming familiar with the school's office for disability services is that they can extend accommodations and modifications that may have been granted during earlier years of education. Many institutions rely on tutoring, extended time on tests, and a quiet environment to complete assignments as primary treatments. It may not be much, but registering with disability services tells the university that each student exists and has unique needs.

Wear disability as a political symbol. Speak loudly about it, and vary your techniques in becoming a full member of campus. Find allies in the lesbian, gay, bisexual, transgender, and questioning communities on campus as they often possess a history of struggle and liberation. Focus on professors who research through lenses of critical theories. Read professors' published bibliographies, looking for topics that speak to progressive educational practices. Seek out staff members who advise groups dealing with social justice. If this does not yet exist, start a learning disabilities club or student group, which could be an exciting way to explore your disability and take pride in differences. Register to give campus tours to prospective students, offering a unique view of our creative abilities to overcome obstacles via nontraditional methods. Also, some universities send undergraduates to high schools to speak to students, and this may be an opportunity to spread the message that learners are unique and to be celebrated, not searched out for remediation. A lecture of this nature may give hope to prospective students who are struggling with inadequate funding for special education and a lack of social supports. This is the message someone should hear, instead of believing that they do not belong in college.

INVESTING IN LEARNING DISABLED STUDENTS

Learning-disabled students can only advance if there is a bridge built by higher education. To do this, universities must provide dedicated resources to learning disabled students when requested. In the university, it is the learning-disabled student who decides when and how to open up, or "come out" about their disability. When a disabled student does come out with needs, universities will be best suited to assist if they already have a relationship with their students. This may take the form of professor-to-student mentoring, or administrative round-tables with cultural groups on campus. Especially important is constant mentorship and assessment by faculty in internships, practicums, and social activities that make sense to learning disabled students (Bejou & Bejou, 2012). This type of investment asks higher education to enter into democratic camaraderie with their students instead of servicing them as "customers." A deep relationship of this type will keep them in the classroom and close to the educators who can influence and change their lives.

Another area of investment is the university assistive technology laboratory and the marketing of that service. My experiences across four universities have run the spectrum from competent programming to a complete disregard for learning disabilities, both in terms of staff and space. In one case, the assistive lab was in the basement of an unrelated building and a special key was needed to enter. Alternatively, I have seen state-of-the-art laboratories with dedicated (and disabled) support staff trained in best practices. These laboratories give structure to the disabled student where they can grow socially and emotionally. If universities allocate funds for supportive labs, students will have the time and space to develop relationships with peer mentors, which could lead to increased retention. Mentoring is the principle variable graduates use to describe high achieving environments leading to graduation. Universities should implement learning disabled-to-learning disabled mentoring and support this initiative throughout their tenure on campus. Sadly, the importance of mentoring relationships is overlooked, as only 22% of universities have such programs (Chambliss & Takacs, 2014).

Universities must also dedicate resources and space to a learning disability professional on campus who has parity with other service providers on campus. This office should be apart from the university counseling center, as disabled services require a license appropriate to psychology *and* education. The most accurate professional would be a school psychologist with experience in treatment planning and consultation with educators. A competent school psychologist specializes in the latest interventions in academic and social/emotional issues. They can also acquire the sensitive and culturally-appropriate instruments used to measure cognitive ability and academic achievement (Vega et al., 2015). I have been affiliated with campuses where these duties were contracted out (creating unnecessary costs to the student) or put upon the counseling staff. Counselors typically work with students gaining insight into adjustment issues, and while a learning disability may be one of them, not all counselors have expertise with disabilities.

Ultimately, universities must invest in the learning disability culture on campus. This disability, often misdiagnosed by professionals, is the invisible taproot for so many academic troubles (Tzivinikou, 2014). Typically, campuses focus on supportive services instead of the causes of disabilities. "Cognitive ramps" need to be built for us to use in discovering who we are and why we are here. These ramps also help higher education see us and our needs (Yalon-Chamovitz et al., 2016). An example of a ramp could be as elementary as a celebration, lecture, or presentation on learning disability and success. It could go so far as college presidents and board members sharing their experience on the topic. Or to have universities invest in labs, staff, and faculty who not only have an expertise in learning disabled education but have a disability themselves. This culture could be promoted by students through aligning with other groups that have struggled for openness and acceptance on campus. The point is not just to be included in a diversity plan, but to be a supported and valued culture on campus. To attain status as a culture, disability must be visible and speak loudly with a recognizable voice.

A VISION

> There is a university where learning disabled students learn, grow, and go on to be of service to society. This institution is varied in its student body, with people from an assortment of cultures and backgrounds. One of these groups is learning disabled, and those students come from a unique and creative place of problem solving and resilience. They add to the university, and the administration holds them in regard. The president and board of trustees are public about taking their counsel as they have come to know and depend on them for their unique perspectives. The university is positively regarded in industry, and the students who make it strong go out into society and change how the world looks at disability.

To create the currently fictional university described above, the learning disabled must liberate themselves from the need to change their fundamental nature into what they believe someone expects. They can learn much by allying with those who have remained true to their culture while becoming visible, such as LGBTQ and minority groups. This is a political fight requiring higher education meeting them and celebrating their cultural recognition on campus. All of this is done by knowing them, funding assistive laboratories, and providing trained professionals who can design unique educational plans for their success.

There are people who say the learning-disabled cannot achieve "at level" and be equal parts of society because of their distinct methods of learning. They point to their difficulty producing work that is similar to a mainstream cohort as evidence of their "impairment." These people subscribe to compulsory able-bodiedness, requiring every person be fit at every moment of life (Jordan, 2013). These people will be disappointed, as that is not part of who the learning-disabled are. But the learning-disabled know these voices, as many of them grew accustomed to years, if not decades, of people in authority telling them that they can't learn like other students. These voices may sound like school counselors, teachers, and families, but they are not the final authority on success.

We are.

REFERENCES

Bejou, D., & Bejou, A. (2012). Shared governance and punctuated equilibrium in higher education: The case for student recruitment, retention, and graduation. *Journal of Relationship Marketing, 11*(4), 248–258.

Chambliss, D., & Takacs, C. (2014). *How college works*. Cambridge, MA: Harvard University Press.

Gibbons, M., Cihak, D., Mynatt, B., & Wilhoit, B. (2015). Faculty and student attitudes toward postsecondary education for students with intellectual disabilities and autism. *Journal of Postsecondary Education and Disability, 28*(2), 149–162.

Greenstein, A. (2015). *Radical inclusive education*. London, UK: Routledge.

Jordan, T. (2013). Disability, able-bodiedness, and the biopolitical imagination. *Review of Disability Studies: An International Journal, 9*(1), 26–38.

Madaus, J. W., Banerjee, M., & Hamblet, E. C. (2010). Learning disability documentation decision making at the postsecondary level. *Career Development for Exceptional Individuals, 33*(2), 68–79.

Martin-Baró, I. (1994). *Writings for a liberation psychology*. Cambridge, MA: Harvard University Press.

McRuer, R. (2006). *Crip theory: Cultural signs of queerness and disability*. New York, NY: New York University Press.

Morgado, B., Cortes-Vega, D., Lopez-Gavira, R., Alvarez, E., & Morina, A. (2016). Inclusive education in higher education? *Journal of Research in Special Education Needs, 16*(1), 639–642.

Oliver, M. (2009). *Understanding disability: From theory to practice*. New York, NY: Palgrave.

Pelkey, L. (2001). *In the LD bubble: Learning disabilities and life stories*. Boston, MA: Allyn and Bacon.

Sparks, R., & Lovett, B. (2014). Learning disability documentation in higher education: What are students submitting. *Learning Disability Quarterly, 37*(1), 54–62.

Tzivinikou, S. (2014). Universal design for learning-application in higher education: A Greek paradigm. *Problems with Education, 60*(1), 156–165.

Vega, D., Lasser, J., & Plotts, C. (2015). Global migration: The need for culturally competent school psychologists. *School Psychology International, 36*(4), 358–374.

Walker, L. (2016). Impact of academic support centers on students with disabilities in postsecondary institutions. *Learning Assistance Review, 21*(1), 81–92.

Yalon-Chamovitz, S., Shach, R., Avidan-Ziv, O., & Rinde, M. (2016). The call for cognitive ramps. *Work, 53*(2), 455–456.

CHAPTER 23

Final Thoughts: Political Struggle in Higher Education

BEN WHITBURN AND CHRISTOPHER McMASTER

Genuine attempts to be inclusive in the present day—to provide educational opportunities to all—must reach farther than those taken so far. Higher education providers must make study options available to not only people with physical impairments, but also sensory, intellectual, developmental, and psycho-social conditions that may manifest episodically. Any number of intersectional identifiers can also impact on a persons' capacity for study, including ethnicity, gender, age, socio-economic context, and citizenship status. Moreover, in the context of increased globalisation and mobility of persons—a field to which country-specific higher education providers enthusiastically work—institutions are expected to be proactively supportive in their response to individual learning needs. Laws have been enacted, and policies have been created, but there is still much more to do.

This struggle is political. Political struggle is what has led to people with disabilities gaining access to higher education institutions worldwide—an agonism that may have commenced in the 20th century, but one that knows no end, and knows no parameter. Throughout history, collective identity has provided the catalyst for challenging exclusionary cultures of higher education through joint mobilisation, most notably in relation to racial inequalities, as well as discrimination on grounds of gender and disability.

In the first edition of this Manifesto, we reminded readers of Ed Roberts, who made history by successfully litigating for admission. It was the early 1960s and Roberts, who became quadriplegic after attracting polio in his teens, took up residence in the Cowell Memorial Hospital for want of accessible lodgings, from which he attended classes. Support at the time was ad hoc, funding precarious, and staff often did not understand their roles and responsibilities to provide Roberts's access to learning. But in the words of a Noble laureate whose musical phrasing regularly references social injustices, inequalities and moral atrocities, the times they were a' changing.

Roberts worked—his attendance forced the university to scrutinise its culture—its own physical environment and its practices. However, this realisation would take collective effort. As Patterson (2012) writes, Roberts was soon joined in Cowell by seven other students with physical impairments. Though segregated in their makeshift home, they created a student hangout replete with poster covered walls, an improvised beer room, and a pool table. Work, for the residents of Cowell, was both intellectual and social. Through ongoing comparison, they soon realised "the remarkable presence of relationships founded on shared experiences of disability" (Patterson, 2012, p. 479). As a group they adopted the moniker the "Rolling Quads", which as Patterson describes, was branded as "a coalition of disabled students determined to increase accessibility across campus, build a residence outside of the hospital, and secure financial assistance for personal care attendants" (p. 480). Successful to this end, the group evolved into an effective political force, a disability rights group that lobbied for the creation of a student support model, the Disabled Student's Program (DSP). The Berkeley example was a forerunner of present-day student support offices at higher education institutions internationally.

Across the Atlantic, similar political actions were taking place. The Union of the Physically Impaired Against Segregation (UPIAS), an organisation formed exclusively by disabled people, published a manifesto of their own in 1976 entitled the Fundamental Principles of Disability. For UPIAS, similarly to the Rolling Quads, the principal cause of exclusion for people with disabilities was not their impairments, but the barriers that prevent them from participating freely in society on par with able-bodied people. It is worth quoting them at large to clarify their sitpoint (quoted in Oliver, 2009, p. 43):

> as a group, we are excluded from the mainstream of social activities. In the final analysis the particular form of poverty principally associated with physical impairment is caused by our exclusion from the ability to earn an income on a par with our able-bodied peers, due to the way employment is organised. This exclusion is linked with our exclusion from participating in the social activities and provisions that make general employment possible. For example, physically impaired school children are characteristically excluded from normal education preparatory to work, we are unable to achieve the same flexibility

in using transport and finding suitable housing so as to live conveniently to our possible employment, and so on.

This manifesto would go on to serve as the departure point for the influential social model of disability—a cultural artefact that has had unmistakable impact internationally. The social model underpins the work of many disability activist organisations throughout the world, such as the Disabled Peoples International (DPI, 2012). Though not specifically concerned with higher education in its development, the social model has found application in numerous pan-national developments, including the United Nations Convention on the Rights of People with Disabilities (2006) (The Convention). The Convention explicitly cites educational inclusion for people with disabilities. Further, individual countries have responded in their own way to these initiatives for developing context-specific inclusive educational systems, which generally cite the social model as underpinning principles (read Rieser, 2008; European Agency for Special Needs and Inclusive Education, 2018).

THE NECESSARY ADVANCEMENT OF INCLUSION IN THE SECTOR BEYOND PARTICIPATION

We are determined to remain optimistic about the future inclusivity of higher education, as the COVID-19 pandemic gradually fades into our memories. Like Read et al. (2023), we advance that current conditions offer a unique opportunity to consider how things might be different for people with disabilities, on the basis that we draw heavily on commanding conceptual ideas like ableism to drive our inquiries, and that we seek out the voiced experiences of those who have experienced it, to consider otherwise. Put simply, ableism is a concept that we can use to interrogate how ability comes to matter, and how this supposedly underpins the conditions within which we live (Campbell, 2009). In higher education, we maintain that such an approach would allow for a more comprehensive conceptualisation of inclusivity: one that goes beyond (but importantly does not leave behind) already successful attempts to widen participation, but also takes steps to improve student success and attainment, the study experience and transition beyond higher education towards equitable employability. Comprehensive expansion of this kind necessarily requires paying close attention to the difference disability can make to the sector, for as Titchkosky (2022, p. *) writes,

> Instead of proceeding with the notion that all is good, reasonable and fair, if it were not for the vagaries of embodied existence, we might ask how institutions such as the University proceed by acting as if disability is absent and we could begin to act as if disability is present and will remain so.

Picking up on Titchkosky's (2022) concern for the status quo of supposed reasonableness, systematising inclusiveness in a post COVID-19 existence might take on several core projects that might start with institutional policies, but whose redesign cannot go without the input of students (and staff) with disabilities. For this reason, we start with big ideas here, before moving to closer disability-oriented approaches chapter authors have themselves contributed to this end. First, a comprehensive approach to inclusive design must surely draw on interrogating how frameworks of competency come to matter to universities in connection to workplaces, if the sector seeks to contribute to necessarily diversifying workplaces (Corcoran et al., 2022). Second and accordingly, how curriculum may be designed in ways that does not necessary appeal to universality, but does do away with the necessity to make individualised accommodations for students with disabilities, cannot go unaddressed (Bunbury, 2020; Pittman & Brett, 2022). Third, necessary reflection on why universities insist on keeping disability away from the concerns of professorial and teaching staff is worthy of interrogation, to ensure they are not complicit in ongoing wilful acts of exclusion (Thomas & Whitburn, in press). Stressing heterogeneous connections here also expands to the interconnections between people, resources, technology and animals that enhances an inclusive imaginary (Goodley & Runswick-Cole, 2016). Fourth and finally, flexibility, much like that which was provided during the height of COVID-19, and that permitted all students to study online or face-to-face, access materials in multiple ways, and submit assessment when possible, might be given more permanence in sector-wide pedagogical considerations, rather than administrative limitations (Dube & Baleni, 2022; Wertans & Burch, 2022).

As was the first edition of this book, this iteration of *Disability and the University: A Disabled Students' Manifesto, 2nd edition* is a clear guide to not only what students want (and need to know), but what higher education providers—whether north or south—should provide in this post COVID world. Each chapter presents a benchmark for students to follow as they travel through the institution, and also lays clear what they should expect. Each chapter is also a clear statement of what every institution of higher education should provide. While every country has its own practice and laws based on its own experience, arbitrary national boundaries should no longer be a reason for practices that do not meet student need. This book speaks across borders, and leaves little doubt about what needs to be done to develop more inclusive teaching and learning spaces in higher education.

REFERENCES

Bunbury, S. (2020) Disability in higher education—do reasonable adjustments contribute to an inclusive curriculum. *International Journal of Inclusive Education, 24*(9), 964–979.

Campbell, F. (2009). *Contours of ableism: The production of disability and abledness.* New York, NY: Springer.

Corcoran, T., Whitburn, B., & Knight, E. (2021). Inherent requirements in higher education: locating You in Us. *Perspectives: Policy and Practice in Higher Education,* 1–7. https://doi.org/10.1080/13603108.2021.1986166

Disabled People's International (DPI). (2012). *Home: Disabled People's International.* Retrieved from: http://www.disabledpeoplesinternational.org.

European Agency for Special Needs and Inclusive Education. (2018). *Inclusive education for learners with disabilities.* Retrieved from https://www.european-agency.org/news/seminar-inclusive-education-learners-disabilities.

Dube, N., & Baleni, L. (2022). The experiences of higher education students with disabilities in online learning during the COVID-19 pandemic. *Journal of Culture and Values in Education,* 5(1), 59–77.

Goodley, D., & Runswick-Cole, K. (2016). Becoming dishuman: Thinking about the human through dis/ability. *Discourse: studies in the Cultural Politics of Education,* 37(1), 1–15.

Oliver, M. (2009). *Understanding disability: From theory to practice* (2nd ed.). Basingstoke, UK: Palgrave Macmillan Press.

Patterson, L. (2012). Points of access: Rehabilitation centers, summer camps, and student life in the making of disability activism, 1960–1973. *Journal of Social History,* 46(2), 473–499.

Pitman, T., & Brett, M. (2022). Disability and Australian higher education: The case for an Accessible model of disability support. *Australian Journal of Education,* 66(3), 314–325.

Read, S., Parfitt, A., Bush, T., Simmons, B., & Levinson, M. (2023). Disabled people's experiences of the Coronavirus pandemic: a call to action for social change. *Social Inclusion,* 11(1), 38–47.

Rieser, R. (2008). *A commonwealth guide to implementing Article 24 of the UN convention on the rights of people with disabilities.* London, UK: Commonwealth Secretariate.

Titchkosky, T. (2022). University inclusion practices–re-encountering the status quo: An interpretive approach. *Journal of Disability Studies in Education,* 1(aop), 1–23.

Wertans, E., & Burch, L. (2022). 'It's Backdoor Accessibility': Disabled students' navigation of university campus. *Journal of Disability Studies in Education,* 1(aop), 1–22.

Whitburn, B., & Thomas, M. K. E. (2022). Ontological assessment decisions in teaching and learning. In *Assessment for Inclusion in Higher Education* (pp. 74-84). Abingdon, UK: Routledge.

Contributors

Katelin Ander is courting PhD programs to continue her work blending disability theory with literary criticism. Katelin examines the way that disability is constructed and viewed through language and metaphor in media across milieus, particularly where these lines intersect with other social divisions. In addition to academic applications of disability studies, Katelin continually advocates for disability-conscious pedagogy in higher education. Katelin is currently based in Idaho, in the United States.

Mostafa Attia is a disabled researcher from the global south. He has contributed to numerous national and international consultancies, all revolving around the concept of inclusion in education, employment or other related disability matters. Mostafa worked as a teaching assistant at the University of Leeds, School of Sociology, where he is completing his PHD in "revolution, global development and disability politics in Egypt." As part of his disability activism in many countries, Mostafa is now chairing a disabled people organization (DPO) in Leeds, as well as being board member to other disability organizations. Mostafa has published a paper to discuss the protection policy for work-family balance and disability in Gulf countries.

Denise Beckwith is a PhD Candidate at Western Sydney University. Denise's PhD is exploring sexual education provision for women with physical disability and potential experiences of violence. Denise has in excess of sixteen years work experience in the disability-rights advocacy sector having exposure to and experience in both non-government and government service provision. She has experience in disability consultancy roles and more recently, has academic teaching experience in the discipline of social work. Denise believes disability inclusion will only be achieved through pro-active consultation.

Matthew Bereza (PhD) is an associate professor of psychology and Latin American Studies at Tiffin University, Tiffin, Ohio. Matt investigates how ecologies and trauma inform our experiences and how we may improve these systems. On campus and in the community, Matt stays active with the Latin American Student Organization and Project Peace. The focus of these groups is to foster understanding, acceptance, and peace within and between people and local groups. When not working, Matt can be found on his motorcycle or trying to get his natural-leavened sourdough formula to produce consistent loaves.

P. Boopathi (PhD) is an Assistant Professor in the Department of English, Aligarh Muslim University, Uttar Pradesh, India. His research interest includes Disability Studies, Palestine and West Asian Literature, Life Writing Studies, Postcolonial and Resistance Literature. For his Doctoral Research, he worked on the identity construction of Palestinians in the life narratives written by Palestinian refugees. Boopathi has published articles in journals, edited books and presented research papers in conferences both inside and outside India in his areas of research. He offers a specialized course titled "Disability Studies and Literature" to final year Master students of English Literature and ELT.

Laura Yvonne Bulk (PhD, MOT) is a daughter, cousin, friend, woman, femtor, Dutch settler, first-generation university student, learner, teacher, Disabled scholar, occupational therapist, and a JEDI activist (justice equity diversity inclusion). She is a Clinical Assistant Professor in Occupational Science & Occupational Therapy and Accessibility Advisor for health professional students at the University of British Columbia on xwməθkwəy'əm Territory. Her practice, teaching, research, and service focus on enhancing belonging, exposing ableism, challenging disablism, exploring solidarities, and moving collectively toward justice.

April B. Coughlin (PhD) is an assistant professor of Adolescent Special Education in the Department of Teaching and Learning at the State University of New York at New Paltz. Dr Coughlin began her career as a New York City public high school teacher. Her research focuses on disability, access, and equity. As a lifelong wheeler, she is committed to increasing understanding and education about the need for physical access and inclusion for individuals with disabilities.

Justin Freedman (PhD) is an Assistant Professor in the Department of Interdisciplinary and Inclusive Education at Rowan University in New Jersey, USA. At age five, Justin was diagnosed with Attention Deficit Hyperactivity Disorder (ADHD) and identified as having a learning disability. Justin formerly taught middle school social studies and high school special education. Justin's research focuses on ADHD, clinical simulations in post-education, and approaches to disability and accommodations that create more meaningful participation for post-secondary students. His research has been published in journals including the *International Journal of Inclusive Education* and *Disability & Society*. Email: freedmanj@rowan.edu

Georgia Geller (PhD, RN) is a Research Fellow and casual academic at four universities across Australia. She also advocates for, and, trains Assistance Dogs in the capacity of Certified Professional Dog Trainer while being an Assistance Dog Handler herself. Areas of research include Assistance Dogs, CALD, mental health and the disability sector. Georgia teaches postgraduate research to inform healthcare practices at Flinders University, South Australia and has published extensively in peer reviewed journals. She is presently working on a legislative audit across Australia related to Assistance Dogs and public access.

Justin Harford is Program Coordinator at Mobility International USA, working to increase the participation of people with disabilities in mainstream study and volunteer experiences between the United States and other countries. Justin is blind. He studied Spanish in Mexico in the summer of 2008 and spent an academic year working on his bachelor of arts in Latin American history at the Pontifical Catholic University in Santiago, Chile. Justin blogged about his experiences at http://yanquireflections.blogspot.com/2010/ and he has written many tipsheets and best practices at www.miusa.org. This is Justin's first volume, and he looks forward to contributing to more in the future.

Jentel Van Havermaet is a PHD candidate in the domain of Disability Studies at the Department of Special Needs Education of Ghent University (Belgium). Her research focuses on the meaning of visual impairment basing on a multilayered postmodern approach and lived experiences. She published an article of a qualitative study on how mothers and fathers living with a visual impairment experience parenthood. She works on accessible participation in conferences, and on a relational understanding of visual impairment through contextualized lived experiences. Jentel can be contacted at: Jentel.VanHavermaet@ugent.be

Leechin Heng (PhD) completed her doctorate at the University of Canterbury. The focus of her study is to explore the meaning-making of inclusion in an initial teacher education programme in Aotearoa New Zealand. Her research interests include disability studies, inclusive education, discourse analysis, among others. In addition to the current volume, Leechin has contributed two other book chapters: *Belonging, Rethinking Inclusive Practices to Support Well-Being and Identity*; and, *Who's In? Who's Out? What to Do about Inclusive Education*.

Laura Jaffee is a fifth-year doctoral candidate in Cultural Foundations of Education with a concentration in philosophy of education. She has certificates of advanced study in Women's and Gender Studies and Disability Studies. Her research interests include disability justice, anti-imperialism, the role of U.S. universities in supporting U.S. empire, and political movements in education. She is also committed to labor justice and supports the efforts of graduate workers fighting to unionize. She previously worked in an elementary school in Minnesota.

Neera R. Jain (PhD) is Senior Lecturer at the Centre for Medical and Health Sciences Education at the School of Medicine, Waipapa Taumata Rau The University of Auckland in Aotearoa New Zealand. Neera has been advancing access to health professions education since 2007, variously as a disability resource professional, researcher, and educator. She co-authored *Equal access for students with disabilities: The guide for health science and professional education* (Springer Publishing, 2020) and *Accessibility, inclusion, and action in medical education: The lived experiences of learners and physicians with disabilities* (AAMC, 2018), along with other publications. Her anti-ableist research agenda activates critical disability studies theory to advance justice in medical education.

Travis Chi Wing Lau (PhD) completed his PhD at the University of Pennsylvania and is a postdoctoral teaching fellow in English at the University of Texas at Austin. His research interests include 18th- and 19th-century British literature, the history of medicine, and disability studies. He currently serves as an editor for *The Deaf Poets Society* and as a referee for *Review of Disability Studies*. His academic writing has been published *Digital Defoe, Disability Studies Quarterly, English Language Notes*, and *Romantic Circles*. His creative writing has appeared in *Wordgathering, Assaracus, The New Engagement, The Deaf Poets Society, Up the Staircase Quarterly* and *QDA: A Queer Disability Anthology*.

George Low (PhD) is a researcher in social justice and inclusion. He gained a doctorate in Education from the University of Edinburgh and explores the issues faced by disabled people through the lived experiences of musicians who have a physical impairment. As a wheelchair user and musician George has a special interest in attitudes and perceptions towards disabled people with a focus on disabled musicians in particular. George lives in West Lothian with his wife Jeanette and his assistance dog, Fogle.

Rod Michalko is teaching Disability Studies in the Equity Studies Program of New College, U of T. He is an adjunct faculty member in the Department of Sociology and Equity Studies, OISE, and also participates in the Critical Disability Studies Program at York University. Titchkosky and Michalko have jointly authored five books and numerous articles in disability studies.

Karen McCall (MEd) provides strategic planning, consulting and training on accessible content design and inclusive education. Karen has been an advocate for a global inclusive education standard since 2009. Her experience as a leader in the field of accessible content design includes participation in the following committees: ISO 32000 (PDF), ISO 14289 (PDF/Universal Access), Technical Standards Committee for Plain Language and Technical Standards Committee for ICT, both part of the Accessible Canada Act. Her latest research, "Rethinking Alt Text to Improve its Effectiveness," was published in the Springer Lecture Series "Computers Helping People with Special Needs", July 2022.

Christopher McMaster (PhD) is the author of *Educating all: Developing inclusive school cultures from within* published by Peter Lang. He is the creator and lead editor of the *Survive and Succeed* postgraduate student support series, with editions published in the UK, USA, Australia, New Zealand, South Africa and Scandinavia. Christopher has recently been an Assistant Professor of Education, Special Education at Augsburg University, Minneapolis, USA. He has since returned to his adopted home of New Zealand where he teaches in a local special school. He writes both fiction and non-fiction, including seven novels, two anthologies of short stories and poetry, and has edited collected fiction works. Christopher's latest academic book is *Radical Behavior: Humanizing the Functional Behavior Assessment (FBA)*. His author website is: www.christophermcmaster.com

Amanda Müller is Associate Professor and researcher in the area of Assistance Dogs for disabling conditions, ranging from issues of laws and policy to handler experiences. Dr Müller lectures in postgraduate nursing, population health, and epidemiology. She is a nationally accredited Assistance Dog trainer and behaviouralist.

K. Muruganandan (PhD) is an Assistant Professor at the PG Department of English, Thiruvalluvar University Constituent Arts and Science College, Kallakurichi, Tamil Nadu, India. Areas of his research interest include disability studies, Tamil studies, cultural studies, translation and sociology of literature. He worked on the politics of Shakespeare in colonial Tamil drama for his PhD, and has coedited a book on literature and human rights. Muruganandan has published in journals and presented papers in seminars in the fields of his research interest. He is presently working on the disability rights movements in South India.

Mike Oliver (PhD) obtained his BA (Hons) Sociology and Social Anthropology at University of Kent in 1975 and his PhD in 1979. He then worked as a lecturer at the University until 1982. In 1991 he became the first Professor of Disability Studies in the United Kingdom at the University of Greenwich and worked there until his retirement in 2003. He co-founded the international journal *Disability and Society* and was an executive editor until his retirement. He was an internationally recognised academic and political commentator, having participated in several major policy reviews in education, health and social services and published numerous books and articles on disability and other social policy issues over the last 30 years. He has also made many appearances on national and regional television and radio. He was an active member of the disability movement and worked with many organisations of disabled people.

Erin Pritchard (PhD) is a lecturer at Liverpool Hope University in the department of Disability and Education. Her research focuses on the social and spatial experiences of people with dwarfism within the built environment. Her work engages with Geographies of disability and Geographies of body size to understand how particular spaces are exclusionary for people with dwarfism. More specifically, her work explores how people with dwarfism navigate through different spaces and negotiate both social and spatial barriers, including unwanted attention. Her work has appeared in *The Scandinavian Journal of Disability Research* and *Geography Compass*.

Maree Roche is a postgraduate student in Inclusive Education at Deakin University, Melbourne Australia. She is an advocate and writer in mental health with her research focus on the learning experiences of secondary school students with mental health challenges. Maree is also an award-winning visual artist who expresses her lived experience with bipolar disorder through a variety of creative mediums. Maree tweets @MareeRoche.

Beth Rogers has a BA in News-editorial journalism from the University of Illinois. She holds a Masters degree in Medieval Icelandic Studies from the University of Iceland. She is now pursuing a PhD at the University of Iceland exploring the cultural significance of dairy products in medieval Iceland. She also holds an MA.Ed and has taught English, Computer Science and a variety of other subjects in the US, Taiwan and Iceland. Currently, she is a monthly contributor to

Medievalists.net and its affiliate, *The Medieval Magazine*, and host of the Medieval Icelandic Sagas podcast.

Katie Roquemore is a fourth-year doctoral candidate in Cultural Foundations of Education with a concentration in Disability Studies at Syracuse University. Her research interests include the experiences of disabled students and teachers in elementary and secondary schools, including how policy impacts those experiences. Her current research is working toward making teacher education programs more inclusive of disability in both curriculum and in who is admitted as a future teacher. She taught high school English before pursuing doctorate studies.

Tafadzwa Rugoho is an adjunct instructor/part-time lecturer at Great Zimbabwe University and a doctoral candidate at the University of KwaZulu-Natal, where he is specializing in participation of persons with disabilities in empowerment initiatives in Zimbabwe. He holds an MSc in development studies and an MSc in strategic management. He has vast experience in disability issues, having worked in the field for more than ten years. He has authored a number of journal papers and book chapters. Tafadzwa is also a disability activist.

Fady Shanouda is a doctoral candidate at the University of Toronto at the Dalla Lana School of Public Health, in the Social and Behavioural Health Sciences division. His doctoral research focuses on improving access to learning for marginalized groups, especially disabled and mad students in higher education. Fady has published scholarly articles in the fields of Disability and Mad Studies and has explored topics in history, education, resistance, activism, and material culture. Fady is also a course instructor at the University of Toronto and at Ryerson University teaching introductory and advanced courses in Mad Studies.

Zoie Sheets is a current Masters of Public Health student at the University of Illinois at Chicago (UIC), focusing on health policy and health outcomes for disabled populations. As an incoming medical student at UIC, Zoie is also highly interested in how physicians are taught (or not taught) about disability. She has served as the chair of several student disability committees at UIC, both during her undergraduate and graduate years. In her work for The Inclusive Collective campus ministry, Zoie examines how faith spaces can be both physically and culturally accessible for disabled people.

Yosung Song (PhD) is an Assistant Professor in the Education Department at Moravian College, U.S.A. She is a former elementary teacher in South Korea as well as a former member of the graduate student organization, Beyond Compliance Coordinating Committee (BCCC) at Syracuse University, U.S.A. With

BCCC members, Yosung worked to create inclusive campus environment and increase campus accessibility for students at Syracuse University. Her research interests include the implementation of inclusive practices to support diverse students in schools, especially students with refugee or immigrant backgrounds. Email: songy@moravian.edu.

Tanya Titchkosky is Professor of Disability Studies and Associate Chair of OISE's Social Justice Education Program at University of Toronto. Other research areas include: Interpretive methods; phenomenology as informed by Black studies; critical indigenous studies, queer and feminist theory; sociology of knowledge.

Hetsie Swartz Veitch is a fourth-year Fulbright Foreign Student in Cultural Foundations of Education at Syracuse University. Her PhD research critically explores disability in South African higher education. She considers the intersection of race and disability embedded in the discourse of disability in policy frameworks and institutional practices at South African universities. Hetsie's tenure as head of disability support services at a well-known South African university urged her to center the lived experiences of disabled students in her work. She will return home to South Africa to advance disability studies scholarship and research after completion of her PhD.

Ben Whitburn (PhD) Lectures in Inclusive Education at Southampton University, United Kingdom, in the undergraduate and postgraduate teacher education programs. Ben has published a body of literature in the field of disability studies in education that explores, in particular, how knowledge on disability translates to policy and practice in diverse educational contexts. In addition to the current volume, Ben has edited *Postgraduate Study in Australia: Surviving and Succeeding* alongside Christopher McMaster, Cat Murphy and Inga Mewburn (Peter Lang). Ben tweets @BenWhitburn.

Megan Zahneis is a student at Miami University in Oxford, Ohio, United States, studying journalism and disability studies. She is a member of the national board of DREAM (Disability Rights, Education, Activism and Mentoring), part of the National Center for College Students with Disabilities, and co-founded her school's Students with Disabilities Advisory Council. In that role, she has aided in the creation of a model accessible classroom and a disability cultural space on her campus. Megan regularly presents on the student experience of disability and serves on the executive team of a conference for high school students with disabilities. She tweets @MeganZahneis.